BUILDING A UNIFIED AMER
HEALTH CARE SYSTEM

BUILDING A UNIFIED AMERICAN HEALTH CARE SYSTEM

A Blueprint for Comprehensive Reform

GILEAD I LANCASTER, MD

Foreword by Congressman Jim Himes
Foreword by David L. Katz, MD, MPH

JOHNS HOPKINS UNIVERSITY PRESS | *Baltimore*

Johns Hopkins University Press

2715 North Charles Street

Baltimore, Maryland 21218

www.press.jhu.edu

Library of Congress Cataloging-in-Publication Data is available.

ISBN 978-1-4214-4588-5 (paperback)

ISBN 978-1-4214-4589-2 (ebook)

A catalog record for this book is available from the British Library.

Special discounts are available for bulk purchases of this book. For more information, please contact Special Sales at specialsales@jh.edu.

The difficulty lies, not in the new ideas, but in escaping from the old ones.
—John Maynard Keynes

CONTENTS

When I was sworn into Congress in January of 2009, the epic political battle over the passage of the Affordable Care Act was just over the horizon. For a political newbie, the next year was a baptism by fire. Explosive town hall meetings were interspersed with excruciating forays into the intricacies of drug pricing policies, visits from practitioners of every conceivable medical specialty, and story after devastating story of constituents unable to purchase expensive drugs or denied health insurance because of having had breast cancer.

One thing was clear. Our health system, while capable of nearly miraculous care, was serving far too few people at far too high a price. And its unfathomable complexity and inefficiency were hurting nearly everyone involved. But because health care is so deeply personal to people, and because one man's inefficiency is another man's paycheck, the forces arrayed against change were ferocious.

The histrionics at health care town hall meetings in 2009 included charges that "Obamacare" was a radical overhaul of the health care system, a full-blown government takeover set to install "death panels" that would gleefully deny grandma lifesaving care, sparing her the horror of living in a country running apocalyptic deficits. Red-faced and profane "Tea Party patriots" promising me political extinction were matched by besuited lobbyists representing every facet of the "Medical Industrial Complex" opposing the reform or making sure that their financial interests were undamaged. Hastily assembled dark money flooded the media with ads designed to terrify Americans. I was bewildered one morning to see on television that I was planning to vote to provide erectile dysfunction drugs to child molesters.

Fortunately, before my election, I had come to know a thoughtful and unassuming cardiologist named Gil Lancaster. Gil had taken an interest in the hulking superstructure of the system in which he worked and began to serve as a sort of spirit guide to me through its many bewildering complexities.

Gil instantly saw that the promises of catastrophic devastation delivered by a socialist takeover were nonsense. In fact, Gil recognized that the Affordable Care Act was a relatively light-touch reform of the *health insurance* market that made only incremental changes to the actual business (and cost) of providing Americans with health care.

The legacy of the Affordable Care Act was to decrease markedly the number of uninsured Americans, by some 20 million people, to forbid the devastating practice of "underwriting" whereby Americans with preexisting conditions such as asthma or diabetes were refused coverage by insurance companies, and to make Medicare coverage less expensive to senior citizens. Most if not all of these changes were fully "paid for" by increases in taxes on the highest-income taxpayers.

As laudable as these achievements were, Gil's fears were realized. Very few changes were made to the embedded complexity, inefficiency, and spiraling costs of the underlying system. The benefits of the reform were often lost on consumers facing consistently rising insurance premiums and deductibles. Medical practitioners continued to burn time and money arguing with insurance companies and Medicare.

This frustration led Gil and a group of his colleagues to develop the EMBRACE proposal, the subject of this book. In conversation after conversation over many years, Gil and I fell into a familiar pattern: he would draw on his medical experience to offer what *should* happen, while I would draw on my political experience to offer what *could* happen.

The EMBRACE proposal, and the background and context provided in this book, offers the most lucid and straightforward diagnosis and cure for the pathologies of our health care system I have encountered in over a decade of public service. You don't need to agree with every aspect of the proposal to recognize the elegance with which it addresses the critical objective we must have for health care: that it provide universal access to high-quality care at an affordable price. Even those who take issue with EMBRACE should read Gil's comprehensive diagnosis of the problems it seeks to solve. This book should be read by my colleagues of both parties, their staffs, and the many thousands of public servants with a role in the health care system.

As I have told Gil many times, the chaos that roiled the passage of the Affordable Care Act makes me skeptical of the possibility and likelihood of fundamental, rather than incremental reform. There are tectonic forces at play that will not simply disappear. Critically, inefficiency is in the eyes of the beholder. Hospitals, which are sometimes characterized as untransparent centers of excessive cost, are also in many instances a municipality's largest employer, to be defended at all costs by mayors and legislators. Pharmaceutical companies are attacked for their profitability even as some of their cash flows go into the development of miracle drugs and vaccines.

Consumers, of which I am one, also have contradictory desires. Nothing is more toxic in political discussions of health care than the word "rationing," conjuring, as it does, denied care and death panels. The reality, of course, is that every valuable product and service since we hunted and gathered on the plains of Africa has been rationed by some mechanism or another. Belief to the contrary notwithstanding, health care in America is rationed. It is rationed passively by arbitrary and regressive factors such as whether you are employed, live in a rural or urban area, or are wealthy or poor. It is rationed actively by insurance companies, which explains a great deal of the vitriol sent their way. Wherever you are on the political spectrum, it's hard to manage what you can't really talk about. Dr. Lancaster takes this third rail of health benefit coverage head on and proposes a mechanism to apportion public spending based on evidence-based need yet allow continued access to all remaining health care services through commercial insurance.

Finally, the institution in which I serve, the US Congress, jealously guards its powers and perquisites. A good portion of any Congress's energy is spent tinkering with Medicare and Medicaid, "guiding" research at the National Institutes of Health and the Department of Defense, and otherwise channeling the hubbub of constituents' concerns and aspirations into the health care system. Gil offers the Federal Reserve, an institution both chartered by and insulated from Congress, as an analog for a decision-making entity that might be guided more by science and evidence than by the enthusiasms of legislators. It is a useful and interesting analogy to help guide Congress as it considers a more comprehensive approach to health care reform. But as a practitioner of retail politics, I know that constituents care more intensely and viscerally about the price and availability of the drugs they buy and the doctors they see than they do about the details of health care system administration.

These challenges, and many more like them, can be overcome. At some point, there may be no choice. The Medicare system, which provides insurance coverage to senior citizens, has an unfunded liability—promises made to those current and future seniors, but not yet paid for—of $55 trillion, a figure almost twice the current national debt. Households and businesses continue to pay an increasing portion of their paychecks for insurance premiums, deductibles, copays, and other medical expenses. This is likely unsustainable, and as economists point out, unsustainable things tend to stop.

The immense value of Gil's contribution to the debate, apart from its lucid diagnosis, is that it offers a roadmap out of our quagmire. The EMBRACE endpoint may not be precisely where the economic, cultural, and political pressures land us. It's important to remember that our peer nations, places like Germany, the United Kingdom, and Japan, have different systems that combine the public and private sectors in varying ways. All of them, incidentally, achieve better aggregate health outcomes than the United States, with dramatically lower per capita expenditure. To move in a better, more efficient direction, over whatever time frame is required, will require a sense of the destination. Dr. Lancaster has offered one of the best roadmaps to those desired goals.

FOREWORD
David L. Katz, MD, MPH

Among the repeated frustrations of my career in public health, and my lived experience for that matter, is the human tendency to argue over trees while missing the forest. There are innumerable examples, but medical marijuana serves well as both a vivid and widely known illustration.

There was intense debate in the United States about the legalization of medical marijuana. To be clear, this was not the larger debate about legalization in general, for recreational use. This was the debate about legalizing the use of a drug by prescription, under physician supervision, for limited and specific therapeutic indications.

Were the ferocity and duration of societal debate on this topic a matter of the drug's toxicity? Certainly not. Many drugs vastly more toxic have long been legal for medical use. Most of the agents referred to collectively as "chemotherapy" are among the entries here, as are a diversity of others.

Was the debate concerning addictiveness? Again, clearly not. Both prescription drugs, such as the sedative class of benzodiazepines, and tobacco are more addictive and more dangerous. Here, too, the list extends to many other entries.

The resistance to medical marijuana seemed to be all about the fact that a given compound was already "illicit," and thus should stay that way. Looking beyond that trivial tautology, however, would have revealed an opportunity to get at far more meaningful principles. A debate raged over medical marijuana, cocaine—yes, cocaine—was already legally in medical use. I know this in more than the abstract, having used a cocaine solution any number of times during my years as an emergency physician to treat epistaxis, a severe nosebleed. This was a long time ago, and also concomitant with the medical marijuana debate. I vaguely recall a wry roll of my eyes over the frivolous medical marijuana debate each time I accessed that routinely available therapeutic solution of cocaine to help stop a patient's nasal hemorrhage. While on this particular rant, it's worth noting that while heroin, derived from morphine, is illegal, dilaudid—also derived from morphine and roughly five times more potent than heroin—is in every hospital pharmacy.

These are just illustrations, and there are many more. We have a penchant, it seems, for making rules without making sense. We readily tangle ourselves up in a Gordian knot of superficial concerns, while neglecting true fundamentals. In any given domain, we depend on some clear-minded thinker to sever that knot, clear the path, and invite us to begin anew.

In the area of health care coverage, Dr. Lancaster is just such a person. He is not claiming erudition in health economics; he is not a policy wonk. He is, instead, a clear thinker, with a perspective informed by many years of doing what health care coverage is supposed to be about: caring for patients.

Like the medical marijuana debate, the health reform debates that have roiled American politics for decades are stunningly blinkered. For example, is health care a right, or a privilege? The oxygen, ink, and electrons allocated to that fraught question would be hard to tally, but in my view, Dr. Lancaster cuts through all of that with the exact right answer: yes. In other words, it can be either; it depends.

Consider, for instance, the mangled and bleeding victim of a hit-and-run accident, an innocent pedestrian mowed down on a crosswalk. Would any decent soul require proof of insurance before rendering treatment in this scenario? In such a situation, care is rendered no matter the ability to pay, and rightly so. Care is rendered to an often unconscious victim who cannot be consulted for consent, or dissent. Care is rendered as if it were a basic human right. And so it is. At the extremes, where life or limb is in imminent and addressable peril, we as a culture handle health care as a right. Basic decency requires no less of us, and we all seem to accept that.

But as noted, there is a spectrum in play here. At its other extreme are discretionary, and perhaps even at times frivolous interventions couched under the rubric of medical care, but not actually treating a medical condition. Purely cosmetic varieties of surgical body sculpting come to mind. Basic decency would not require that all of us be entitled to the latest sensation abuzz in Hollywood at our fellow taxpayer's expense.

And, of course, there is the inevitably more challenging expanse in between. There are, as well, those times when treatment of an individual is actually of more good to the body politic than to their own body. A facile example of this is the widely encouraged practice of vaccinating young children against SARS-CoV-2 to better protect the vulnerable adults they might encounter.

Imagine a system where health care is treated as a right when it is a right, and as a privilege when it is a privilege. Now imagine adapting responses to also suit the expanse in between, so that what should be accessible without barrier is; what warrants a personal burden of cost has one attached. And, imagine that for public goods the principles of behavioral economics are thoughtfully leveraged.

Dr. Lancaster's imagination got there ahead of ours, and he has appended to it years of work elucidating the relevant details. Those of us first brought together by Dr. Lancaster years ago to develop the EMBRACE construct believe, quite simply, that health care policy should make sense. Were we starting from scratch and devising a system to pay for medical care, we would be unlikely to propose anything so ham-handed as one-size-fits-all choices. Dr. Lancaster invites us here to begin again, as if everything—even completely sensible solutions—were in play.

In this book, Dr. Lancaster, the originator of this simple, elegant, powerful, and once you think about it, rather obvious approach to health care coverage, makes his detailed case. It is a case that honors sense and science, basic principles and edge cases, personal responsibility and public good, and honors the lore of American-style individualism into the bargain.

Health care coverage can be fiscally responsible, and compassionate.

Reimbursement can be respectful of both personal responsibility and public good. Health care across a spectrum of services can be both a human right and a privilege. If you *embrace* these fundamental principles, then you have just the right resource in hand for an insightful and illuminating read.

There really is a better way. If enough follow where Dr. Lancaster has spent years leading, perhaps we could actually get there from here.

ACKNOWLEDGMENTS

Like many physicians practicing in the United States, I have always been struck by the problems entrenched in our health care system that daily affect my patients and colleagues. But like most of my physician and nursing coworkers, I had believed that health care reform was beyond my expertise or scope of practice. These were matters that seemed to be better handled by lawmakers and health policy experts.

After experiencing many attempts at "health care reform" by these experts, it dawned on many of us in the medical field that maybe we needed a different approach. In my case it started with the help of Drs. Kimberly Yonkers and Charles Landau as we formulated over dinner many of the concepts of what we would later call EMBRACE.

Within a few months, interest grew among our colleagues, which led to many interesting and productive discussions that eventually resulted in the decision to publish our proposal. Thanks to the help of coauthors Ryan O'Connell, David Katz, JoAnn Manson, William Hutchison, Charles Landau, and Kimberly Yonkers, and advisers Harlan Krumholz and Sherry Glied, the plan was finally published in the *Annals of Internal Medicine* in April 2009.

Unfortunately, by the time the proposal was published, most of the attention around health care reform had shifted to what was soon to become the Affordable Care Act. EMBRACE, like other reform proposals, became sidelined.

During this time, through my involvement with the American College of Cardiology's Board of Governors and Health Affairs Committee, I learned the importance and difficulty of advocating Congress for our patients and our profession. I especially want to thank Dr. Thad Waites, the chair of the ACC's Health Affairs Committee as well as

Nick Morse, Lucas Sanders and the rest of the committee's team. What I learned on the committee, as well as during our annual legislative meetings and our visits to congresspeople and senators on Capitol Hill, was invaluable.

I also want to thank Congressman Jim Himes, who showed an early interest in our health care reform approach. In the years since we first discussed EMBRACE in 2008, we have had several productive discussions that have significantly advanced its content and helped formulate some helpful advocacy strategies.

My interest in writing this book was prompted by the COVID-19 outbreak. The pandemic categorically exposed the dysfunction of the American health care system and brought out the need to separate health care from politics.

The book would not have been possible without the help of Dr. Joseph Drozda. Over the two years that it took to write it, Joe acted as a consultant, collaborator, editor, and friend. Even though we belong to different ends of the political spectrum, we almost always agreed on what is needed in health care reform. Our collaboration is a testament to the idea that the practice of medicine has no political affiliation and that it is feasible to run a health care system free of politics.

Finally, I want to especially thank my wife, Mary Dale, for her constant support and patience. For over a decade she has endured my passion for health care reform and has been a part-time widow for the past two years while I was writing this book. It is this support through thick and thin that has allowed me to pursue this passion. Thank you!

BUILDING A UNIFIED AMERICAN
HEALTH CARE SYSTEM

Introduction

Even before the COVID-19 pandemic began in 2020, the US health care system was already showing signs and symptoms of ill health. One clear sign was the large number of attempts to reform it and one clear symptom was how ineffective and inefficient the system was at delivering health care to the American public.

More than any other developed country, the United States has been grappling for decades with how to provide health insurance to its population, especially its most vulnerable. But the COVID-19 pandemic has made clear that the problem isn't just of how many Americans have insurance; it is also the challenge presented by an archaic and decaying infrastructure rooted in the twentieth century that is not prepared to take on the challenges and demands of a modern, science-based health care system.

In this respect, most approaches to health care reform have neglected the true causes of the system's dysfunction, namely its lack of a unified infrastructure and oversight. Instead of addressing these "big-picture" issues and tackling root causes, lawmakers have found it easier to nibble around the edges and focus on a few of the most evident problems (like the number of uninsured or the use of preexisting conditions by insurance companies to deny coverage).

Physicians know that a systemic disease like diabetes can affect many organs. They can treat the heart, eye, and kidney diseases that the diabetes has caused in a patient, but they know that until they can effectively control or cure the diabetes, these treatments will be less effective, and the organ problems will continue.

It is therefore not surprising that it took a group of physicians (and other health care professionals) to recognize that the US health care system suffers from a "systemic" disease. Consequently, the group endeavored to address underlying problems the same way they might treat a systemic medical condition: with evidence-based solutions.

This group of nonpartisan health care professionals believed that discussions of reform needed to address the broader more pernicious problems and be led by health care professionals rather than by politicians, insurance companies, and partisan thinktanks. With the aid of health care economists, public health experts, and lawmakers, the group ultimately developed a holistic health care reform proposal that they called EMBRACE (**E**xpanding **M**edical and **B**ehavioral **R**esources with **A**ccess to **C**are for **E**veryone). Their proposal was first published in 2009 in the *Annals of Internal Medicine*. Over the past decade, the plan has continued to evolve and improve. This book presents the latest version of EMBRACE.

It needs to be understood that the comprehensive discussions about the health care system covered in this book involve a whole host of disciplines. These include, but are not limited to, public health, economics, history, health policy, public finance, information technology, and even banking reform. All are robust academic fields in their own right but are seldom discussed together when considering health care reform, as in this book. This presents a unique opportunity not only to explore these varied disciplines but also to see how they might work together to find new solutions for what has been a vexing problem.

Banking and financial reform is not often identified with health care system restructuring. Yet the examination of the politics around the creation of the Federal Reserve is a particularly important aspect of the EMBRACE proposal. Although it was not the first to propose a semi-independent medical board based on the Federal Reserve,[1] the plan is the first to fully integrate it into a holistic vision for health care system reform. For that reason, this book will provide added focus on the historical and political parallels between the banking and financial turmoil of the early twentieth century and the current situation in the American health care system, and what we might learn from such parallels.

Of course, when dealing with this number of wide-ranging disciplines it is not possible to do justice to all the potential contributions of each. Instead, this book endeavors to extract the important elements of each field and demonstrate how they can be coordinated in a cohesive health care reform solution. The intent is not to present an exhaustive dissertation on the state of the American health care system, since that has been covered quite well by others,[2,3,4] but rather to explain the need for its across-the-board reform.

Although this book is evidence-based, it is written for a broad readership who may not have a background in the many disciplines that are covered. Wherever possible, the book provides references to the supporting documentation that are accessible on the internet to assist the reader in further exploring the complex issues that surround American health care.

CHAPTER 1

The American Health Care System Disorder

Anyone who believes the US health care system is actually a system has not worked in it, been a patient in it, or tried to reform it. Although there have been tremendous advances in medical and surgical therapies over the past century in the United States, these have occurred in the setting of a health care delivery infrastructure that is ever worsening, replete with inefficiencies, bureaucracy, inequality, profiteering, and politics.

American health care is a system where patients are referred to as "consumers" and are often regarded as a commodity by insurance companies when they contract with doctors and hospitals. It is a system where doctors and hospitals have to spend money and many hours dealing with insurance companies; not to improve the quality of patient care or treatment outcomes but rather to receive payment for services in a game that serves to increase profits for the companies and their shareholders. It is a system where outcomes such as infant mortality and life expectancy are worse than in other developed countries, while the cost of care is more than twice as high. It is a system where not having insurance is a risk factor for bad health, death, and even bankruptcy. And it is a system where access to health care is dependent on one's age, income level, prior military service, employment status, and even ethnicity.

The most vital (and most troubling) issues with the current health care system in the United States are its ineffectiveness and inefficiency. Its *ineffectiveness* is reflected in the most important indicator of any health care system: its outcomes. In 2017 the Organisation for Economic Co-operation and Development (OECD), representing the top industrialized countries in the world, reported that the United States ranked at the bottom of the three clinical outcome measurements they follow. The United States ranked 34th (out of 36 member countries) in maternal mortality, 32nd in infant mortality, and 27th in longevity or life expectancy.[1] At the same time, per-capita cost, the big-picture indicator of a health care system's efficiency, showed that the United States spent more than any other country in the OECD—more than twice that of most of the other members.

How this ineffective and inefficient "system" came to be is a long and complicated story best described elsewhere. What is clear is that there was never any thought of design or structure to the developing system. It has evolved into a complex landscape of private and public insurance schemes with little oversight and few rules. In many ways, it is the perfect product of free-market capitalism and Americans' distrust of their federal government. Additionally, the health care infrastructure is still rooted in the horse-and-buggy days of the early twentieth century and has simply not kept pace with the increasing sophistication of clinical care, primarily because there is no compelling economic reason for third-party payers to change their approach.

To best understand how to fix this system, I think it is important to spend some time to better understand its entrenched complexity.

Complexity of Health Insurance in the United States

The majority of we "consumers" think of health insurance as something that covers our doctors' visits, hospital stays, and medicines. But in the eyes of US health policy, each of us is a part of a larger group based on what kind of insurance we have and who pays for it.

The US health care system has evolved to include three main categories of health insurance: a publicly funded insurance system (either by federal or state governments), a system of private (also referred to as commercial) insurance, and the insurance system for veterans.

Let's first look at the publicly funded system. The majority of our public health care system is overseen by the Department of Health and Human Services (HHS). This government body oversees three health insurance programs and several agencies. Sometimes it appears that the criteria for who the three public insurance programs cover were chosen arbitrarily: (1) Medicare insures individuals who are 65 years old or older and also those who have a recognized disability; (2) Medicaid insures those with a low income and those who are minors (typically under 18 years of age); and (3) Indian Health Service (IHS) provides health services based on one's ethnicity (only Native Americans are covered).

In addition to insurance program oversight, HSS administers agencies, including: the Food and Drug Administration (FDA), which oversees drugs and medical devices; the Centers for Disease Control and Prevention (CDC), which oversees much of the nation's public health; and the National Institutes of Health (NIH), which funds most US medical research that is not sponsored by drug or device companies.

Despite all of these insurance programs and health care agencies being under the direction of HHS, Congress funds (or earmarks) each separately, resulting in long and acrimonious political arguments. Importantly, this process makes it very difficult for HHS to develop cogent long-term plans or strategies.

Another publicly funded but independent health care agency is the Veterans Health Administration (part of the Department of Veterans Affairs), which offers health coverage based on a person's military service history. It is also funded separately by Congress.

And then there is our private health insurance system.

Despite the perception that "private health care" is a single entity run by private insurance companies, it is significantly more complicated. Over the years, private insurance providers (more accurately referred to as commercial insurance firms) have developed various organizations, networks, and programs—health maintenance organizations, preferred provider organizations, exclusive provider organizations, clinically integrated networks, health care exchange programs—not for better patient care, but rather as profit-making entities or as responses to regulatory/legislative pressures. Each of these schemes often has its own set of patients, its own set of providers, its own set of hospitals, and its own set of rules, making them mini autonomous health care systems within a system that generally lacks any oversight.

As a physician, I have come to view these mini systems as tumors, some benign and some malignant, growing within our system. Like tumors, each of these schemes is a self-serving autonomous entity whose only purpose is to grow (and make a profit). This growth is often at the expense of other parts of the health care system—such as the poor or unemployed—which in turn is bad for the overall health of the overall health care system.

One illustration of this is the practice of many commercial insurers of preferentially enrolling patients who are at a low risk of requiring expensive medical care (which, after all, is their business model). Even though this was significantly reduced by the Affordable Care Act's provision that insurers cannot discriminate on the basis of *preexisting conditions*, they have many other mechanisms of "risk profiling" their potential enrollees.

An example is the frequent practice of making it more difficult (and more expensive) for smokers or other "high risk" groups to be enrolled. This leaves these higher-risk persons more likely to be uninsured and subsequently more likely to forego preventive care. This, in turn, increases the chance that these uninsured patients will later end up needing expensive care for heart disease or cancer, which could have been prevented if they had had preventive care through insurance. This not only increases the cost to the overall system but also negatively impacts the global health of the system—much like a malignant tumor.

In Figure 1.1, I have attempted to capture the complex interactions of the various components of US health insurance. The circle labeled Public/HHS represents the public components of the system overseen

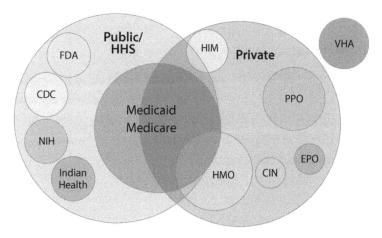

FIGURE 1.1. The US health insurance structure. See main text for details and abbreviations.

by HHS and containing the CDC, the NIH, the FDA, Medicare, Medicaid, and the IHS.

The circle labeled Private represents the landscape of private/commercial insurance. It contains many schemes: health maintenance organizations (HMO), preferred provider organizations (PPO), exclusive provider organizations (EPO), clinically integrated networks (CIN), and health insurance marketplace (HIM).

The smaller circle on the right labeled VHA represents the relatively independent Veterans Health Administration, which is so independent from the rest of our system that it might as well be in another country.

This diagram also attempts to show the chaotic interactions that have developed between commercial and public insurance systems. More than half of Medicare and Medicaid have become privatized (through systems called Medicaid managed care and, euphemistically, Medicare advantage) while HMOs, which started off as strictly private insurance programs, have started to include Medicare and Medicaid patients. And, under the Affordable Care Act (also known as Obamacare), which stipulated the creation of marketplaces for private insurance (HIMs), many of these commercial plans are publicly subsidized.

Complexity of the US's Health Care Delivery (and the Corporatization of Health Care)

The way health care is delivered to patients in the US is also extremely complex and chaotic and to a great extent is driven by the equally chaotic payment system. In general, patient care takes place in an "outpatient" setting, in a hospital (often referred to as "inpatient" care), and in extended care facilities.

In the past, "outpatient" referred to the setting in which patients received care for minor ailments, for preventive therapies, and for follow-ups after inpatient treatments. Inpatient care was usually reserved for patients with acute conditions that required rapid evaluation or intensive treatment. Operations and most procedures also traditionally took place in hospitals, as did chemotherapy, substance detoxification, and even rehabilitation services. For the more long-term patients, such as those needing long-term rehabilitation and memory care, there were chronic care facilities such as nursing homes.

These categories were not unique to the US health care system, but over the years, financial/insurance incentives and pressures brought on by the advent of Medicare (especially privatized Medicare) and HMOs have changed the meaning of these terms. Many procedures and therapies that were once considered to be inpatient procedures, are now done in "outpatient surgical centers," while some patients in hospital emergency rooms are considered "outpatient observation patients." There is no evidence-based health advantage to these categories, they are used as a payment scheme and are purely reactions to insurance pressures.

Insurance pressures have also changed the physician-patient interaction. Traditionally, doctors were in charge of running their medical practices, setting their prices, and charging the patient according to the service rendered. In the long-ago era of Marcus Welby, physicians could open a solo outpatient private practice office and know that insurance would cover their patients' visits and services with a minimum of red tape. This allowed the clinician to spend as much time with the patient as needed.

But over the years, private insurance companies began to increase their demands on practices. One example is a practice known as "prior authorization." This is the process of having to get approval from the patient's insurance company before a test or procedure is performed. Prior authorizations arbitrarily second-guess physician decisions based on frequently dubious scientific evidence. They also reduce the efficiency and increase the cost of patient care by requiring physicians to spend time getting authorizations or hiring someone to do it. It has been estimated that these burdens add $150 billion a year to the health care system, the cost of which is mostly handed down to the physician's practice, and ultimately to the patient.

There were also pressures from commercial insurance companies on physician practices to join larger practices and accept only patients with certain insurance plans. More recently there have been new insurance company-induced financial pressures to sell private practices to hospitals, thus making administration-heavy hospitals responsible for both inpatient and outpatient services and making physicians their employees.

The growth of HMOs after the Health Maintenance Organization Act of 1973 has also significantly contributed to the corporatization of outpatient medical practices. Although the intent of the law was to foster the growth of not-for-profit organizations vested in the good health of their members, it quickly led to the development of for-profit companies that hired physicians as employees on salaries that were linked to reductions in high-cost specialty services and to primary care "productivity" goals. These goals are focused more on cost savings than on clinical outcomes or patient satisfaction. This cost-reduction focus benefits HMO shareholders and unfortunately impresses lawmakers as a potential model for sustainable publicly funded programs.

The original HMO concept (also termed "prepaid group practice") was envisioned as being physician led. The for-profit model, although in actuality representing nothing more than redesigned health insurance, retained the physician integration approach either through contracting or direct employment. This transformative concept—that insurance companies can (and some think, should) run medical practices—was a seminal change in how the public and lawmakers understood health care delivery in the United States and has changed the focus of health care leadership from health care providers to insurance providers.

As outpatient practices have changed over the years, US hospitals have also undergone significant transformations. There was always an extraordinary diversity in the types of hospitals, including medical-school affiliated academic hospitals, community-based not-for profit hospitals, "public" (also sometimes called charity) hospitals, hospitals for veterans, religiously affiliated hospitals, specialty hospitals (for cancer, orthopedics, etc.), and for-profit "private" hospitals. This diversity is quite unique compared to other countries, and has generally been perceived to be an asset of the system, due to the large range of options and increased competition.

However, compared to hospital systems in other countries, US hospitals have the highest administrative costs, which account for about 25 percent—or more than $200 billion—of total hospital costs per year. Administrative costs appear correlated directly with the degree of penetration of "market-oriented payment" (private insurance as opposed to government payers) in the hospital's service area. Countries that primarily use single-payer systems incur half of the administrative costs of US hospitals. This suggests that the reduction of administrative costs in the US would best be accomplished with a simpler and less market-oriented payment scheme.

The incredible variety of hospital types in the US has grown out of its uniquely complex health care system and has both disadvantages and advantages. The main disadvantages of the system are its redundancy and inefficiency. Because of budgetary considerations, some hospital services (such as cardiac rehab programs[2]) are often underrepresented compared with need. On the other hand, more lucrative services (like heart surgery) may be overrepresented. This means that there may be longer waits for the underrepresented services or no availability at all, while the overrepresented services might result in wasted resources due to duplications and even a dilution of experience for doctors and other medical personnel. How would you like to have your heart surgery performed by a surgeon who only does a couple a year?

Because some hospitals, such as those belonging to the VHA or those owned by a particular HMO, are supported by unique financial mechanisms, the patients covered under these programs are limited to participating hospitals for their regular care. This significantly limits the choice and even mobility of the patient/consumer, as there may be only a limited number of participating hospitals.

A rather unfortunate secret is that most American hospitals need to tailor medical care based on a patient's insurance status. Although this might seem unfair and maybe even discriminatory, for the most part, this practice exists for the patient's benefit. If patients lack insurance or have inadequate insurance, they may be unable to afford tests and treatments unless services are carefully managed by the patient's hospital and doctors. Consequently, the care team, which often is different for these patients than for "private" patients, might elect to do testing and treatments in the hospital that might be more appropriate to the outpatient setting. Further, doctors might need to prescribe cheaper, and possibly less effective, medications on discharge.

Because of having to care for uninsured patients, hospitals in poorer areas have more limited funds and therefore are challenged in providing the best services to their patients, even for those who have insurance. Additionally, these hospitals tend to be in regions with sicker populations that rely heavily on hospital-based care, further exacerbating the problem.

In addition, the way that hospitals are paid by Medicaid and Medicare is variable, unpredictable, and mired in politics. This makes it all the more difficult for hospitals to make business decisions and devise future financial plans.

There are, however, some good aspects of the US hospital system, such as the hospitals' community service orientation. Admittedly, much of the stimulus for these programs has come as a result of government-created financial incentive programs.[3] Nevertheless, these programs are helping the communities they serve by addressing what has been termed the social determinants of health. In addition, competition with other facilities often results in better-quality facilities and facility improvements.

The specialized aspect of the US hospital system is not unique. Most industrialized countries have a similar stratified system, from the local "general" or community hospital to the large tertiary teaching hospitals, similar to the Mayo Clinic and the Cleveland Clinic, that may take referrals from all over the country (and even the world). What makes the US system different is that the government runs only a few hospitals (about 20%). More than 90% of hospitals in European countries with some form of single-payer system, such as Sweden and the United Kingdom, are government-run.

Although the merits of government-run hospitals are debatable, in the US there is clearly a public preference for non-government-run hospitals. Much of this is due to the public perception that non-government-run hospitals provide better service and, maybe, better care. Certainly, the 2014 scandals involving VHA hospitals, where dangerously long patient wait times for treatment were allegedly covered up, serve to further that perception. Another common belief is that competition for patients among non-government-run hospitals not only improves service but may also improve the breadth and quality of care.

Over the past few years two major trends have significantly transformed US hospitals. The first is the growth of "health systems," a practice of different hospitals consolidating under a common administrative umbrella. This originally was done in an effort to reduce duplication of services and to lower costs. However, as for-profit groups have become involved, many of these systems have changed their focus, with return on investment and profit seeming to outweigh health care access, quality, and outcomes.

The other somewhat related trend is the almost exponential rise of hospital administrative staff. In the past, the majority of hospital employees were involved in direct patient care, with a small staff of administrators—typically senior doctors and nurses—to help run the day-to-day business of the hospital. With the rise of regulatory, financial, and insurance-related pressures, most hospitals have found the need to hire experts to address non-medical issues. These administrators are trained in the business aspects of health care and are a part of one of the fastest growing professional fields: "health care administration."

This growth of health care administration offers great high-paying jobs to many individuals, and is arguably good for the economy. However, at the same time, it can be argued that these jobs do not provide any direct health benefits to patients or improve medical practice and only drive up the cost of health care without actually improving it. At times, some hospital administrations may even be at odds with the medical or nursing staff based on corporate considerations rather than best clinical practices.

It's not that one can eliminate these jobs and no one would notice. On the contrary, in the current US health care system infrastructure, hospitals and hospital conglomerates would all but collapse without a strong administrative staff (and many have). The issue is that the health care system infrastructure has developed in a way that requires a whole new profession just to navigate through it. Although some of the regulatory hurdles that necessitate health care administrators are concerned with patient or provider safety, most relate to the business aspects of hospital management associated with both private and public insurance.

Complexity of the US Health Care System's Infrastructure

Despite the phenomenal medical, pharmacological, and technological advances in the US over the past 20 to 30 years, the health care system's data and information infrastructure is still deeply rooted in the twentieth century. This deficit is most apparent in the lack of integration into the system of such technologies as electronic medical records, the internet, medical imaging, and health monitoring data. These difficulties stem from the fact that health care data sources grew out of a very different era, when paper charts were used in doctors' offices and hospitals, communication among clinicians was by telephone, "snail mail," and fax, and the results of most testing were captured on videotape, paper, and X-ray film.

The term "electronic medical records" (EMRs) refers to the computerization of patients' medical charts. However, EMRs are much more than just an electronic version of a paper chart. In addition to the documentation of the patient's visit or hospital progress, they include test results, orders for tests and medications, and important information about the patients, such as their pharmacy, their living will, and their insurance carrier. EMRs are also designed to document the provider's service (consult, surgery, therapy, etc.) to support billing the patient or the insurance plan.

However, doctors and nurses often complain of EMRs' lack of user-friendliness, which is likely due to the basic design of most of these systems being focused on maximizing reimbursement rather than on improving clinical efficiency and patient outcomes. Additionally, since these systems are purchased by health care administrators, their designers tend to focus more on features that appeal to health care administration rather than patient care.

A more important impediment is that an EMR from one vendor is often incompatible with that from another vendor. This means that despite the huge amount of information that these EMRs may have about a patient, the information cannot be transmitted to an outside hospital or office unless they have the same system. Instead, the information is sent by mail, fax, or email, the antiquated communication methods they were meant to replace.

This lack of interoperability stems from a lack of coordination of the digital platform, which is actually a group of platforms created by the companies developing EMRs and other software. These companies' business model is based on the proprietary edge their platforms give them rather than on cooperation with other firms to enable interoperability. Although this makes a good business model, it is antithetical to efficient communication among health care professionals and to good patient care.

But this again is not completely the fault of the EMR developers who are simply responding to a diverse and uncoordinated market. Instead, it is due to the archaic organizational infrastructure on which the US health care system is built, and which lacks unified oversight.

Until this infrastructure is changed, it will be extremely difficult to make EMRs interoperable.

The Complexity of Health Care Research in the US

It is fair to say that medical research is one bright spot in the current US system. The list of medical discoveries and inventions (that include chloroform, polio vaccines, Hepatitis B virus vaccine, COVID-19 mRNA vaccines, amongst others) is long and impressive. However, research into how to use some of these incredible innovations at the hospital bedside or in the office, is surprisingly inadequate. The inadequacy of bringing research to the bedside is due to four important factors: misaligned incentives, haphazard priorities, ineffectual implementation, and inconsistent guidelines.

It is no secret that financial profit is one of the key drivers of innovation in our society and is considered an essential element. Dwight D. Eisenhower said, "When shallow critics denounce the profit motive inherent in our system of private enterprise, they ignore the fact that it is an economic support of every human right we possess and without it, all rights would disappear." But the profit motive is often at odds with the goals of a functional health care system—to deliver affordable evidence-based care to everyone.

Misaligned Incentives

The problem is not necessarily in the concept of profit itself but in its misaligned incentives. When a pharmaceutical firm increases the price of an old essential medicine on which it has a monopoly or blocks the use of a generic medicine that might compete with one of its branded drugs, the results are good for the company's profit but not for patients and the health care system. On the other hand, if there were incentives to develop new or considerably improved therapies (especially where there are none currently), pharmaceutical firms would take Benjamin Franklin's advice to "Do well by doing good."

Do we need to spend $112 billion a year[4] to treat psoriasis, a relatively benign skin condition that affects the quality of life of about 2%–3% of the US population? In comparison, care for diabetes, which affects 25%–33% of the population and is the seventh leading cause of death in the US,[5] costs $237 billion.[6] In a society that has unlimited funding, there would be no dilemma about allocating money from private and government insurance programs to support development of therapy for conditions that affect quality of life. But, when there is such a huge profit incentive from increasingly expensive insurance coverage, with little direction regarding priorities, the result is the development of 12 different biologic medicines (treatments that target specific areas of the immune system) from 12 different drug companies to treat psoriasis.

This "me too" phenomenon of multiple drug development for the same condition is very common in the health care marketplace, and has a long history in medical care. It might make sense in other markets where like products drive down prices through competition, but in the health care marketplace, where insurance pays the bulk of the costs, there is really no price competition at the level of the patient/consumer.

In addition, a good deal of the innovation that pharmaceutical firms use to develop proprietary drugs (medicines for which they have a patent, and can control the price) comes from publicly funded research. A recent study found that all 210 drugs approved in the US between 2010 and 2016 benefitted from publicly funded research, either directly or indirectly.[7] Taxpayers contribute through public university research, grants, subsidies, and other incentives. This means people are often paying twice for their medicines: through their tax dollars and at the pharmacy. Yet, there is no clear policy on which of these drugs is worthy of public money.

Haphazard Priorities

These haphazard priorities of research and resources are a result of the lack of a grand design for the US health care system. There is no such grand design because there is no single oversight body that can analyze the need for research and therapy in the health care system as a whole. In the absence of this oversight, pharmaceutical and device companies decide what therapies to develop based on consumer demand (that is divorced from product value because the patient is shielded from the full price) and on profit rather than on public health needs.

Most of the money that pharmaceutical and device companies spend on research is aimed at getting the treatment to market. According to the FDA, this form of *clinical* research consists of 4 phases of development:[8]

Phase 1: Researchers test an experimental drug or treatment in a small group of people for the first time. The researchers evaluate the treatment's safety, determine a safe dosage range, and identify side effects.

Phase 2: The experimental drug or treatment is given to a larger group of people to see if it is effective and to further evaluate its safety.

Phase 3: The experimental study drug or treatment is given to large groups of people. Researchers confirm its efficacy, monitor side effects, compare it to commonly used treatments, and collect information that will allow the experimental drug or treatment to be used safely.

Phase 4: Post-marketing studies, which are conducted after a treatment is approved for use by the FDA, provide additional information including the treatment or drug's risks, effectiveness in broader patient populations, and best use.

It is important to understand that for most potential therapies, funding for the *clinical* phase of research comes from the pharmaceutical or device company. This usually means a very substantial investment in research that may end up showing that the new medicine or device is of no benefit or even may be harmful.

Most phase 3 studies compare the efficacy and safety of the new therapy against what is considered the "standard of care" treatment in order to demonstrate therapeutic *equivalence*. Companies rarely have to demonstrate that the new therapy is significantly better (and safer) than other similar therapies—a type of research that is often termed "comparative effectiveness." Because of this, we often see situations in which multiple (often expensive) medicines are on the market with little information to assist the physician in deciding which one might be better for their specific patient.

Using the biologic treatment of plaque psoriasis as an example, we know that the 12 FDA approved medications are safe and effective, but how do we know which is the best? Because each phase 3 trial may be designed differently, with different patient populations and different endpoints, one cannot reliably compare the data between trials to get an idea of comparative effectiveness and safety. The only way to get this information is through direct head-to-head studies, which are very expensive, not required by the FDA for approval, and rarely done by drug companies. The few head-to-head drug trials that do take place are usually supported with public funding and often compare only inexpensive generic medications because of pharmaceutical company resistance to the inclusion of their branded products in the comparisons.

It is important to understand that the ultimate aim of all this research and development (from the laboratory to FDA approval) is to inform clinicians and patients regarding the effectiveness and safety of medications and devices used in care. Although this information is vital, it is surprisingly hard to come by.

Ineffectual Implementation

Over the past two decades there has been a growth of what are called "clinical guidelines" (CG) and more recently, "appropriate use criteria" (AUC). CGs were developed in the hope of helping clinicians translate research generated information into best practices in the care of their patients. These "evidence-based" recommendations ranged from the utility of diagnostic tests to the best therapies for specific patients.

Unfortunately, almost all of these CGs were, and still are, based on information derived from research studies that were not designed to answer the specific clinical question for which that particular guide-line is developed. Instead, those who compose guidelines are often forced to extrapolate conclusions from data that were collected on different types of patients from those more commonly seen at the bed-side or office. The data used by guideline developers are from studies that were designed for drug approval, not for clinical practice. These studies often limit the age, pregnancy status, coexisting conditions, and risk factors of the patients who are included in them. Excluding these patients allows the drug or device company to get the biggest "bang for the buck" and keeps them safe but leaves guideline devel-opers needing to infer (or make an educated guess) how drugs and devices might perform in patient groups that were not included in the industry-sponsored trials.

So, what do CG developers do about the missing data or about con-ditions or therapies that do not have good studies? They are often left to make educated guesses in these as well. The guideline term for this process is "expert opinion." In the world of science-based guidelines, expert opinion is considered the least reliable form of evidence and is very often later found to be wrong. Yet, many—if not most—CG rec-ommendations are based on expert opinions.

Ideally, there would be a mechanism for systematically capturing and updating the information needed to make more reliable CG rec-ommendations either by recommending or by actually commissioning studies for that purpose. Unfortunately, this is very difficult to accom-plish in the current system because the organizations that usually de-velop CGs don't have the ability to do either.

In the United States, most CGs are developed by specialty or sub-specialty medical organizations. These organizations, which generally represent physicians and clinical care associates (nurse practitioners, nurses, technicians, etc.), are mostly independent of the pharmaceu-tical and device industry, but often do rely on their financial support for many of the organizations' non-academic activities. Also, because there is no overall supervision or coordination of the CG process, CGs produced by individual societies are often developed independently of other organizations' CGs, even if there is overlap. Most of the time the result is that the organizations' CGs make similar recommendations, but occasionally the recommendations conflict. And because there is no umbrella entity providing oversight, there is no process for reconciling the differences.

To complicate matters, there is another type of guideline that has become more prominent in recent years, the AUC. AUCs were loosely based on CGs, and originally were developed by insurance companies to optimize (some might say, limit) the use of certain expensive tests and procedures, such as nuclear stress testing and implantable cardiac defibrillators, and they are employed as part of the prior authorization process. When used in this fashion and applied to individual patients, AUCs lack clarity and have a very heavy emphasis on cost reduction (euphemistically termed "cost effectiveness"). Finally, each insurance company has developed different AUCs, making it difficult for the clinician to know the rules in advance.

In response, the medical societies that had previously developed CGs began also to produce AUCs, with the intent of making them more evidence-based and uniform across insurance companies and of easing the compliance burden on clinicians. Unfortunately, and as with CGs, the lack of data made it difficult to make many recommendations based on anything better than "expert opinion."

However, the most problematic issue regarding CGs and AUCs is how to make them "user-friendly" and allow them to be easily accessible at the bedside or the office. The major limitation to this kind of use is the difficulty that busy clinicians have in learning all the various CG and AUC algorithms. Clinicians also face the question of what to do when CG and AUC algorithms disagree, or when there are multiple CGs or AUCs for each condition. Finally, CG and AUC developers face the challenge of producing timely updates to keep up with ever-evolving science.

The overriding concerns with the deluge of CGs and AUCs is the lack of a single entity overseeing the process. Ideally, this entity would prioritize and commission the development of evidence-based guidelines that include best clinical practices and cost effectiveness considerations and be integrated into practice in a way that it would be clear and user friendly.

The Complexity of Health Care Politics

When meeting with the nation's governors at the White House soon after his inauguration, President Donald Trump started his discussion about health care by saying, "Now, I have to tell you, it's an unbelievably complex subject. Nobody knew health care could be so complicated."[9]

The truth is that it isn't health care that is complicated, it is the politics surrounding health care in the US that is complicated. Left to their own devices, health care professionals mostly agree about what needs to be done, and how to do it. There may be occasional disagreements on the evidence for or ethics of various treatments, but these are usually resolved through science-based or ethics-based discussions.

But in the US, there are many ways that politics enter the practice of medicine. The most obvious is our public health system. Both the heads of the Department of HHS and the United States Department of Veterans Affairs (VA) are cabinet-level positions. This means that the leaders of these organizations answer directly to the president of the United States.

In the case of the VA, the department oversees all aspects of veteran affairs, not just veterans' health, so it is important to have someone who has experience in all aspects of veterans' affairs. But what about HHS? What are the important attributes for heading the public health agency? When he was nominated for the position of HHS secretary in November 2017, the *New York Times* described Alex Azar's background as follows:

> In addition to his experience as a pharmaceutical executive, Mr. Azar brings to the job impeccable credentials as a conservative lawyer. A graduate of Yale Law School, he was a clerk for Justice Antonin Scalia on the Supreme Court in the early 1990s and spent two years as a young lawyer working for Kenneth W. Starr, the independent counsel who investigated President Bill Clinton.

These may be good credentials for a conservative special prosecutor or federal judge, but what makes Mr. Azar qualified to run America's public health care system? What does he know about public health, health care research, health insurance, health care delivery or, most importantly, how to deal with health care emergencies, such as a pandemic?

Surprisingly, Mr. Azar's qualifications for HHS secretary are not much worse than most of his predecessors. Of the 23 secretaries of HHS since the agency was established, only three have been physicians. Most of the others were lawyers, businessmen, and career politicians. This raises what should be an obvious question: If lawyers run the legal system and bankers run the banking system, why aren't health care professionals running the health care system? Why are businessmen and politicians looked to instead of doctors and nurses?

One reason may be that the US doesn't have an infrastructure to support the development of such leadership. As we have previously discussed, the current US health care system has developed as a chaotic collection of private and public mini systems over the past century, with no effective oversight, with HHS growing to fill this void, not by design but by default.

As the oversight body of US public health insurance—such as Medicare and Medicaid—and public health agencies—such as the FDA, NIH, and CDC—HHS's influence in health care delivery has grown as Congress has given it more regulatory power. But HHS's effective oversight of the health care system is limited, since it only has direct influence over the approximately 100 million people that are covered by Medicare and Medicaid (out of a US population of 332 million). The department's influence over some 200 million individuals covered by private commercial insurance is indirect, with the individual insurer having the final say, and its influence over the VHA and uninsured individuals is nonexistent. This means that any HHS policy change or long-term plan applies only to less than a third of the population, and how it might affect the rest of the system is unpredictable.

On the other hand, because they are considered a huge and robust part of the economy, commercial insurance companies, pharmaceutical firms, and medical device manufacturers also exert a huge amount of political influence. Over the years, insurance companies have increasingly been promoting the concept that they are their own health care systems, causing some political leaders to view these privately run systems as a political alternative to a "public" health care system. This in turn has led to the "privatization" or attempted privatization of many public insurance programs like Medicare, Medicaid, and even the VHA.

The conflict between private and public insurance doesn't end there. Although the Affordable Care Act (ACA) increased the number of insured, it also significantly increased the politicization of health care. In addition to asking states to expand Medicaid, the ACA also established the concept of HIMs. These were places where consumers could buy private health insurance in what was hoped to be an "open market," a market that was originally proposed to include both private and public insurance (the "public option") competing for customers based on cost and quality. The Public Option Act would have allowed all citizens and permanent residents to buy into a public Medicare-like program. This federal health insurance plan would have been financed entirely by premiums without government subsidy.

Progressives supported a public option as an alternative to the for-profit health insurance industry, with expectations that it would control costs, promote competition, and prompt delivery reforms and lower provider charges through the bargaining power of a large government payer. Conservatives as well as private insurers opposed the plan because of the implied increased role of government and fear of competition with not-for-profit insurance that would favor the government. Ultimately, the public option failed as a result of many factors, including lack of support from moderate and conservative Democrats, opposition from Republicans and health care interest groups, and ultimately an absence of strong support from the White House.[10]

Another provision of the ACA, that has since been reversed by Congress, was its "individual mandate" provision. This feature was an incredibly important aspect of the momentous reform bill and its annulment threatens its continued viability. To understand why it is so important we first need to understand the important insurance concept of risk pooling. This is where the pooling of consumers with a lot of health problems together with those that are relatively healthy allows the higher cost of covering the unhealthy to be offset by the relatively lower costs of covering the healthy. The more healthy people one has in the pool, the lower the potential payout (or liability) that the insurance provider has. Risk pooling is paramount to the business model of all health insurance concerns. For-profit insurance companies focus on recruiting healthy consumers and minimizing the number with health problems in order to charge competitive premiums while maximizing profits for the company and its shareholders.

Until the ACA, one of the most common ways for the insurance companies to reduce risk was to exclude people with preexisting conditions from the risk pool (or to significantly increase their premiums). Insurance companies recognized that people with certain preexisting conditions would be more likely to need medical or surgical services. When the ACA took away exclusion of people with preexisting conditions as a method for risk pooling, the industry looked to another provision of the ACA to make risk pools financially viable—the individual mandate.

The individual mandate stipulated that everyone in the United States, no matter their health, must own (and pay for) health insurance. From the big-picture viewpoint of public health, this not only would have guaranteed universal health insurance coverage but also would have spread the risk among participating insurers and protected them from adverse selection, that is, covering a disproportionate share of individuals at high health risk. Unfortunately, this meant that many young, healthy people were forced to buy insurance plans that they did not want and were unlikely to use. If they chose not to buy insurance, they would have had to pay a fine.

As *popular* as the abolition of preexisting conditions was in the ACA, the individual mandate was equally *unpopular*. Soon after the ACA became law, the individual mandate was taken to court. In 2012 the US Supreme Court ruled that the mandate was constitutional, but Congress passed the Tax Cuts and Jobs Act in December 2017, which eliminated the individual mandate penalty.

For the insurance industry, the loss of these two forms of managing risk pools meant that there were few incentives for them to join the HIMs, which were such an essential part of the ACA. This, in turn, has led to an increase in the number of uninsured and an increase in premiums and out-of-pocket costs for those with insurance.

But perhaps the most blatant example of the politicization of health care was seen during the early months of the COVID-19 outbreak in the US, when President Trump announced the formation of his task force. The task force was described as a United States Department of State (yes, Department of State, not Department of Health and Human Services) task force that "coordinates and oversees the Administration's efforts to monitor, prevent, contain, and mitigate the spread" of COVID-19.

President Trump appointed Vice President Pence and Secretary Alex Azar to oversee a response to the epidemic. According to the president, Mr. Pence's qualification was being Indiana's ex-governor, while Mr. Azar's qualification was being HHS secretary.[11] Although there were physician advisors, including Anthony Fauci and Deborah Birx, it was clear from the start that the task force was more concerned with politics and the economy than with public health. It was also evident that the president had little interest in following Dr. Fauci's advice, and soon Dr. Fauci was all but fired from the task force. At the same time, public statements from the CDC regarding preventive measures were blocked or heavily censored.

The Complexity of Health Care Reform

When one considers the complexity of health insurance, health care delivery, health care system infrastructure, health care research, and the politics of health care in the United States, one can better appreciate why it has been so difficult to achieve meaningful health care reform. The current US health care system infrastructure is a result of decades of unfettered and rudderless growth and legislation, leading to a gargantuan and incomprehensible structure.

Soon after the passage of the ACA, the Republican members of the

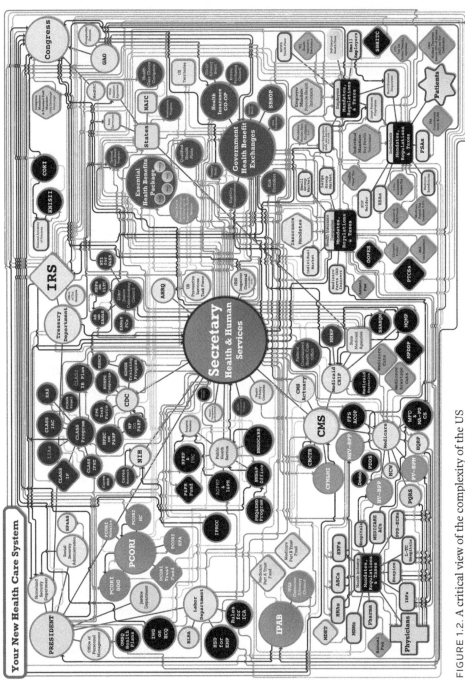

Your New Health Care System

FIGURE 1.2. A critical view of the complexity of the US health care system. The Joint Economic Committee, Republican Staff, modified by author. Original at: https://www.jec.senate.gov/public/_cache/files/8e6dbf02-ca3a-4abe-9de4-a190c43b5c8/obamacare-chart-high-resolution.pdf.

Joint Economic Committee came out with a chart that they called "Your New Health Care System" (see Figure 1.2).[12] Although it was created as a partisan attempt to mock the ACA, it does make a more objective point that the US health care system is extremely complex, even chaotic. It shows the complicated and often ill-defined interactions of the various components of the system. And it also begs the question: If we want to reform this system, where do we start?

Do we pick one, two, or three areas to reform, as was done with the ACA and most other efforts, and hope these reform actions will cause the right combination of interactions to produce the desired results, without incurring the almost certain unintended consequences? This focused strategy has been the pattern followed by policy-makers over the past few decades, not because it is effective, but because it is the only option short of a complete overhaul of the system. This is true not only with the ACA (and the various proposed updates and fixes) but even with the various "Medicare for All" proposals that have been put forward.

Medicare for All would definitely take commercial insurance out of the picture (or at least significantly reduce its influence in the organizational chart). But it would not really change the fact that Medicare and the other public insurance plans would still be significantly susceptible to pressure from political and special interest groups. In fact, since Medicare is overseen by HHS and HHS is part of the executive branch, Medicare for All effectively would be overseen by the president. This might lead to a host of unintended consequences that would change as often as presidents change.

It is time to acknowledge that what we have been promoting as health care reform has not worked and will never work unless we begin thinking outside of the box and more holistically. Maybe it is time to consider completely replacing the system as we know it and rebuilding it from the ground up. Although this sounds drastic, I beg the reader to hear me out and consider a sweeping reformation of our health care system.

If we do decide to completely replace the system, what do we choose to replace it? Ideally, we want a system that is *not* rooted in a federal government beholden to political interests, or run by commercial insurance beholden to financial interests. Ideally, it would be run by a body led and run by health care professionals, independent of both political and commercial interests.

But there are so many other items that we would want on the wish list for this new system. Items that have been so difficult to get in our current system. We will discuss these in the next chapter.

CHAPTER 2

The Ideal American Health Care System

A Wish List

Progress is the realisation of Utopias.
—Oscar Wilde, "The Soul of Man Under Socialism"

Given the opportunity to design a new health care system for the United States from scratch, what should be included in the list of "must-haves"?

This is a vital question to ask because it helps focus on what it might take to achieve the fundamentals of this new system. Many groups, including those representing patients, physicians, politicians, and even insurance companies, have put out statements of "principles" for health care reform. These often reflect the general values and needs of the various groups but rarely include any details. This lack of details has made it difficult to concentrate on how to achieve these aspirations. So, it is important for us not only to list our wishes but also give details.

Here is my wish list: My new health care system must have universal coverage, allow universal access, be user friendly, be effective (with good outcomes) and efficient (with modest public expenditures), be science based, be technologically advanced, allow for free market innovation, have independent oversight, and be run by health care professionals. Also, this new system should allow for those particularly American attributes such as customer-friendly service and minimal government involvement. In what follows are the details.

Universal Coverage

First, I would like to define what I mean by universal coverage, because the term has been used quite loosely. To me, universal coverage means that every man, woman, and child residing in the US is *automatically* covered for *basic* health care services for *no charge*. By automatically, I mean that coverage would start at birth or at the first visit to a health care provider and would continue throughout a person's life. By basic health care services, I mean all lifesaving, life-sustaining, and preventive services that are so essential to all of us. And by no charge, I mean that there would be no physician or hospital bills, no insurance premiums, no deductibles, and no co-payments.

As we saw in Chapter 1, health insurance coverage in the US is as variable and as chaotic as our disordered health care system. Even those who are lucky enough to get insurance from their job or who are eligible for "public" insurance such as Medicare or Medicaid, must go through a complicated enrollment process, make some difficult coverage decisions, and pay various charges such as annual premiums, deductibles, and co-payments.

Others must purchase insurance from the health insurance marketplace (sometimes called the health care exchange program), a process that has proven to be extremely complicated and time-consuming. It is also a process that often has few choices and is quite opaque as to the features of the offered plans.

And then, of course, there is the 10.9% (as of 2019) of Americans who are uninsured. The uninsured often face unaffordable medical bills when they do seek care.[1] In 2019 uninsured nonelderly adults were more than twice as likely as those with private coverage to have had problems paying medical bills in the past 12 months. These bills can quickly translate into medical debt since most of the uninsured have low or moderate incomes and have little, if any, savings.

The experience during the COVID-19 pandemic further drove home the point that for life-threatening conditions and afflictions, having complete coverage is not an option—it is essential. My wish would be that every man, woman, and child residing in the US would be covered *automatically* for *basic* health care services at *no charge*.

Universal Access

Having universal coverage does not guarantee universal access. The limitations of access in the current health care system go far beyond insurance coverage; access also depends on age, income status, employment status (and who your employer is), military service, and ethnicity.

As awareness rises of the racial inequities in law enforcement in the US, it is important to remember that there is also a long-standing ethnic disparity in the US health care system. In 1966 Martin Luther King Jr. observed: "Of all the forms of inequality, injustice in health is the most shocking and inhuman."[2] Some of these disparities are blatant, like having a separate "Indian Health System" for ethnic Native Americans, while other discriminations are more insidious.

One example of the subtle forms of inequality arises from the differences in insurance plans. It is an unfortunate fact that many doctors and health care facilities do not take Medicaid, because Medicaid pays the provider significantly less (sometimes 60% less) than Medicare or commercial insurance. Since Medicaid recipients are more likely to be people of color, the result is a predominant racial inequality to access.

Another source of limited access is the practice of most commercial insurance plans of creating "provider networks," where they limit which providers (doctors and hospitals) their clients can use without paying a "penalty" or even the complete bill.

However, one of the most important sources of limited access is the US tradition of employer-based health insurance. According to recent data from the Kaiser Family Foundation, about 156 million Americans, or around 49% of the country's total population, receive employer-sponsored health insurance (also called group health insurance),[3] making it the predominant source of coverage in the country.

Whatever advantages there might be from having employer-based insurance, the disadvantages are many. For the employer, there are the fees and personnel needed to manage the program, while for the employee, there are co-payments, deductibles, and out-of-network penalties. Employers have also been passing progressively increasing shares of premium payments to the employee while offering plans with fewer benefits.

More importantly, having an employer-based system also ties employees' health insurance to their jobs. In good economic times this might not be a major issue (except that the employee has to change insurance every time he or she changes jobs). But during economic downturns this could be a disaster. This was brought to light during the COVID-19 pandemic, when up to 12 million people lost their employer-based insurance (as of August 2020).[4] This occurred when people needed their health insurance coverage the most and made the impact of getting infected much worse, even if it was not fatal.

People without insurance coverage have worse access to care than people who are insured. Three in ten uninsured adults in 2019 went without needed medical care due to cost. Studies repeatedly demonstrate that uninsured people are less likely than those with insurance to receive preventive care and services for major health conditions and chronic diseases.

My wish would be that every person would have the same access to providers and services. There would be no out-of-network penalties or other limitations to the individual's choice of physicians, hospitals, or other medical services.

User Friendly

What is a "user-friendly" health care system? It is a system free of bureaucratic hurdles for both patients and their providers. Currently, the US health care system has myriad encumbering rules and procedures for both patients and their doctors. Every patient visit requires a ritual of paperwork, insurance verification, and co-payments. Hospital visits are often followed up by unexpected bills for services that were not covered by insurance. There are often supplemental fees and deductibles, and bills from various providers such as pathologists that the patient may never have seen.

Health insurance and billing horror stories affect millions of patients. An illustrative, albeit extreme, example occurred early in the COVID-19 pandemic. In June 2020, the *Seattle Times* reported on a 70-year-old man named Michael Flor, who at the time was the longest-hospitalized COVID-19 patient. Because he made an unexpected recovery, he "was jokingly dubbed 'the miracle child.'" In many ways, this is a testament to the great care that he received for what was then a new and seemingly unpredictable disease.

But when Mr. Flor got home, he received a 181-page itemized bill from the hospital that came to over $1.1 million—earning him a new moniker, "the million-dollar baby." There were charges for the special room he required, for the breathing machine that helped him when his lungs failed, and for each of the medications that he was prescribed during his stay.

As journalist Danny Westneat detailed:

> Flor was in Swedish Medical Center in Issaquah with COVID-19 for 62 days, so he knew the bill would be a doozy. He was unconscious for much of his stay, but once near the beginning his wife Elisa Del Rosario remembers him waking up and saying: "You gotta get me out of here, we can't afford this."[5]

Fortunately, Mr. Flor was covered by Medicare, so it is likely that he would only have to pay a fraction of the million-dollar bill, which in our health care system might earn him another moniker—"Lucky Flor." Unfortunately, many patients are not so lucky and might owe thousands of dollars or even end up in bankruptcy.

My wish is for a system that would eliminate all these little tortures. There would be no charges (or bills) for acute hospital admissions for life-threatening conditions like COVID-19. Office visits would only require a form of identification and charges for hospital visits would be transparent. All basic medical services would be free of charge and any costs for supplemental services would be discussed in advance.

What about the providers? As Medicare and Medicaid grew in size and importance over the past 40 years, commercial insurance companies developed various schemes and business models that helped them compete among themselves and with public insurance. This has led to the creation of a huge bureaucracy that has arisen around the insurers' interactions with health care providers (doctors, hospitals, nursing homes, etc.). There are many bureaucratic issues with the current US health care system, but surprisingly it is significantly more of an issue in the private (i.e., commercial insurance) rather than with the public sector. Each insurer must create its own organizational infrastructure, which generally mirrors that of their competitors, and each has to create its own provider contracting and administrative processes. The bottom line is that the individual clinician or hospital is essentially working in multiple health systems at the same time, resulting in the need for large administrative staffs to keep all the rules straight and to comply with the requirements of these various systems.

This is most apparent with the process of prior authorization. Each insurer has its own prior authorization process and its own criteria for approving (or not) the requested service.

In an ideal health care system, physicians and other health care professionals would not have to get prior authorizations for procedures or testing, and billing would be automatic. There would only be one set of rules that would be based on good scientific evidence promulgated by one health care governance body led by health care professionals.

Additional burdens on the medical practitioner are the constant requirements to keep up with the latest medical developments as well as maintaining their own credentialing. Although this is true with other professions, such as law, the rate of new developments in medical knowledge and technology necessitates constant education and testing.

I will use one of my colleagues as an example. He is an interventional cardiologist in a busy private practice affiliated with a moderately large inner-city community hospital. Like so many other cardiologists, he has also been trained in echocardiography and nuclear cardiology. To maintain his ability to practice in all the fields he was trained for, he must complete a long list of tasks. The most basic of these tasks is maintaining his license to practice medicine. Licensing for all professions is usually done by the state and requires the doctor to show that he or she has taken the required amount of CME (continuing medical education) courses and paid the required fee.

In the distant past, a license to practice medicine was all that was needed. But in 1933 the American Board of Medical Specialties (ABMS) was established with the aim of providing a rigorous process for the evaluation and certification of medical specialists. Over the years the ABMS has grown to represent 24 broad areas of specialty medicine.[6] The largest of these specialties is internal medicine. In 1936 the American Board of Internal Medicine (ABIM) was established—under the umbrella of the ABMS—as a 501(c)(3) nonprofit, *self-appointed* physician-evaluation organization that certifies physicians practicing internal medicine and its subspecialties. The ABIM is not a membership society, educational institution, or licensing body. Its sole role is to certify the qualifications of physicians to practice in internal medicine and its subspecialties. Over the years the number of these subspecialty certifications has grown, and the ABIM now offers 21 subspecialty certifications:

Adolescent Medicine
Adult Congenital Heart Disease
Advanced Heart Failure and Transplant Cardiology
Cardiovascular Disease
Clinical Cardiac Electrophysiology
Critical Care Medicine
Endocrinology, Diabetes, and Metabolism
Gastroenterology
Geriatric Medicine
Hematology
Hospice and Palliative Medicine
Infectious Disease
Interventional Cardiology
Medical Oncology
Nephrology

Neurocritical Care
Pulmonary Disease
Rheumatology
Sleep Medicine
Sports Medicine
Transplant Hepatology

It seems logical that there should be some method of assessing competency in the various specialties and subspecialties of medical practice, but the sheer number of them presents a pressing problem to practicing physicians. For example, my colleague, the interventional cardiologist, needed to certify in internal medicine, cardiovascular disease and interventional cardiology. But that was not the end of it: Every 10 years he has to recertify in each subspecialty (but not in internal medicine) by taking a recertifying exam or completing some mini courses and exams.

To make matters worse for my colleague, he also has to take recertification exams every ten years in echocardiography (through a different certifying organization) and nuclear cardiology (through yet another certifying organization). Although taking exams is a pain, each one usually requires only one day. But the preparation for the exam costs a lot of money and demands a lot of time away from one's clinical practice. My colleague's plight is by no means unique (I have four certifications). The more specialized the doctor, the more certification processes that he or she must undertake.

While there are some data that suggest that those who fulfill the criteria and pass the *original* board certifying exam have better clinical performance than those who have not taken or have not passed these exams, there are no such data for the *recertification* process. This fact, added to the significant time and financial commitment needed to keep up with the recertification process, has become an additional burden to the already busy clinician.

My wish would be that medical credentialing and maintenance of competency would be easy and inexpensive, and would not take a lot of the clinician's time away from professional/clinical work. Ideally, there would be only *one* credentialing body and the process would be integrated with physician workflow.

Effective Outcomes and Prevention

There are many reasons for the US's health metrics, such as infant deaths and life expectancy, being consistently ranked at the bottom when compared to other industrialized countries. One of the most important is the lack of emphasis on prevention. It is more comfortable (and cheaper) for a patient to undergo measures that prevent heart disease, than to have bypass surgery because the heart disease has progressed.

It is also the case that there are often many different therapies for the same condition, without good information on which is the best. These leave the doctor having to make decisions on limited data.

My wish would be to have a system that has the infrastructure to use evidence-based methods to promote lifesaving, life extending, and preventive services. A system that is constructed around scientifically validated methods and which has a mechanism to generate more of these clinical data to fill in any gaps.

Modest Public Expenditures (Taxes, Deductibles, and Other Out-of-Pocket Costs)

There is no doubt that one needs to spend a lot of money to get a good health care system. But other countries have excellent health care systems yet pay much less for them than in the US. The key is to have an *efficient* health care system. That is, a health care system that gets the best bang for the buck.

There are many reasons why the cost in the US system is so high, but some of the factors that have been identified are the high administrative costs associated with private insurance, the American predilection for treating advanced disease with expensive therapies and procedures, and the lack of emphasis on preventive care.

When one looks at the OCED countries that have better outcomes and lower costs, some have a single-payer system, but others do not. What they all have, that the US does not, is a unified health care system. A system that incorporates private and public insurance and has one oversight body reduces duplication of services and increases coordination between its various parts.

My wish for an ideal US health care system is that there would be one body with oversight of both private and public benefits (i.e., insurance). This would eliminate the high overhead associated with insurance billing and reduce the bureaucratic burdens on health care providers. It would also improve the coordination between the various parts of the system. The ideal system would have no out-of-pocket expenditures to the patient for basic health care services, and have affordable (and transparent) methods to "upgrade" coverage through commercial insurance providers.

Science Based

A fundamental tenet of medical practice is that medicine is based on science. Despite this, it is difficult to say that the manner in which health care is delivered in the US has much science behind it. This lack is due to three hurdles: the need to "translate" basic science research into clinical practice, the difficulty of developing truly science-based guidelines, and the challenge of finding ways to use guidelines at the bedside or in the office.

There is no doubt that US bench research is world class. *Bench research* is a term for basic science research that mostly takes place in university and pharmaceutical company laboratories. This research is guided by strict scientific standards. The next step is getting these new discoveries out of the lab and turned into specific therapies for use on humans. This is called translational research[7] and is often broken down into two types (or steps): T1 (basic to human) and T2 (human to population). The science behind these is quite rigorous as well, but because of the many variables in human and population studies, it is not as exact as "bench" research. The final hurdle in bringing health care innovations to patients, sometimes referred to as T3, is the dissemination and clinical implementation of the information in a way that is usable at the bedside or in the office. This is most often done through the development of *clinical guidelines.*

While bench, human, and population research may have a good deal of scientific method behind it, clinical guideline development sorely lacks this rigor. First, there is no clear standard for how to develop the guidelines or even what guidelines need to be developed in the first place. There are different groups that develop guidelines, which are often focused on one particular viewpoint. The science on which guidelines are based is inconsistent (not standardized) and there is no method of testing their efficacy (how well the recommendations actually work). More importantly, much of the evidence that is used in guidelines is "expert opinion," which is in fact, not science at all. The reason why many guidelines must rely on expert opinion is that there is a lack of appropriate science to guide the guideline developers. And once guidelines are developed, there is no good mechanism for checking how compliant clinicians are with using them or for testing how their adoption actually affects outcomes.

The process of guideline development sorely lacks supporting science and in the current system is difficult. What is more, if there are gaps in knowledge needed for guideline development, there is no mechanism to commission the necessary studies to fill these gaps. In the current system, most new therapies, whether medicines or devices, are privately developed. The motivation to develop these therapies is their potential to generate revenue and profit and not necessarily their impact on significant health problems.

My wish for an ideal US health care system is that health delivery would be built around science-based guidelines and the guidelines would be specifically designed for health delivery. In fact, it would be ideal if all medical research would be planned and coordinated, from bench to bedside, and would be based on real patient and public health needs.

In an ideal health care system, profits for pharmaceutical and device companies would be *needs-based.* There would be a mechanism to reward desired therapies and testing as well as true health care innovation, while limiting public expenditures on needless or duplicative therapies.

Technologically Advanced

The twenty-first century has seen tremendous advances in technology, from high-speed supercomputers to cell phones. The advances in medical devices have been just as impressive. In addition to implantable devices such as pacemakers, defibrillators, nerve stimulators, heart monitors, and so many others, there has been a tremendous rise in digital technology that helps monitor and diagnose remotely. In addition, there have been remarkable advances in diagnostic imaging, including ultrasound, nuclear studies, X-rays, and magnetic resonance. But as the number of these innovations seem to skyrocket, there is an increasing need to integrate them with patient care. Key to this is the rise in the use of EMRs.

EMRs evolved from what was called a patient's medical chart. Even as late as the first decade of the twenty-first century, the medical chart most often had handwritten (or typewritten) documentation of patient visits along with reports of test results. They were always on paper. Mail and fax were the only methods for transmitting records of patient visits, reports, and images between doctors and hospitals. In the past decade or two, there has been a significant push to move patient charts onto an electronic medium. One of the most important of these efforts was the development of EMRs, but as they have become the standard, several issues have arisen that hamper their achieving their full potential. Among the issues with EMRs are the inability to consolidate the data they generate for meaningful analysis by the CDC and other government health care agencies, and their lack of interoperability.

Currently, both the CDC's network and the TeleTracking system set up by HHS rely on so-called push data, meaning hospital employees must manually enter data, rather than the government tapping into an electronic system to obtain the information.[8] As cumbersome as this process is in transmitting hospital data, the mechanisms for office-based data submission are even less reliable.

Another factor that has significantly hampered the usefulness of EMRs has been the lack of interoperability—a mechanism of moving data seamlessly from one computer system to another. This has come about because different EMR developers have created their own proprietary software that cannot be used by other developers. This situation is similar to the railroad industry before the Civil War: each company had its own company-specific track gauge, so freight had to be constantly unloaded and reloaded onto new trains when moving into a different area. The Pacific Railroad Act of 1863 set the standard track gauge, which is still the same today. We desperately need this type of EMR standard. The HHS Office of the National Coordinator for Health Information Technology (ONC) has been working to achieve this goal for over 16 years with only modest success.

My wish for an ideal US health care system is that all clinical data would be easily accessible for analysis by national public health agencies and that all EMRs could communicate with each other.

Allow for Free Market Innovation

In an ideal health care system, all health care services should be based solely on scientific evidence of their effectiveness and safety. However, in the US, entrepreneurial interests and profit motives often supersede this ideal. The key is to be capable of guiding this innovative business energy in a way that aligns it with the health care system's goal of developing evidence-based medical products where they are needed most; in other words, to get the incentives right. One of the things that makes the US system unique is the prevalence of the entrepreneurial spirit, which can be a tremendous asset in the right health care environment.

My wish for an ideal US health care system is one that guides entrepreneurial incentives to improve the system rather than take advantage of it.

A Health Care System with Independent Oversight, Run by Health Care Professionals

When COVID-19 first appeared in the United States, the media and the public turned to experts like Dr. Anthony Fauci who headed the National Institute of Allergy and Infectious Diseases, Dr. Deborah Birx, the United States Global AIDS Coordinator, and Dr. Robert Redfield, the director of the CDC, to lead the national response to the coming epidemic. However, President Trump soon created the White House Coronavirus Task Force and appointed Vice President Pence to chair it. Drs. Fauci, Birx, and Redfield were appointed as "members" of the task force, but it quickly became obvious that this was a political task force, and the physician members were relegated only to an advisory status. In fact, of the twenty-seven members of the task force only eight were physicians, with the remaining members being mostly politicians, economists, and businessmen.

It was clear from the start that whatever medical advice offered by those who understood public health and medicine was disregarded in deference to political and economic concerns. These included issues about social isolation, wearing masks, and even medical treatments. But these disagreements also carried more significant consequences for the response to the pandemic. There were disagreements about the amount of testing needed, the use of hydroxychloroquine for treatment and even prophylaxis, and the timing of returning to "normalcy."[9]

In another example of how politics trump scientific data in the current system, the Trump administration quietly issued an edict in mid-July 2020 that stipulated that instead of sending all hospital COVID-19-related patient information to the CDC (as is the practice for all infectious diseases), the data had to be sent to the HHS.[8] This effectively bypassed the non-partisan science-based (and more transparent) agency that is set up to handle epidemics and transferred the data to its political overseer.

Although the politicization of health care was spotlighted during the COVID-19 pandemic, it is not at all new. Politics is inexorably entrenched in the US health care system and most of the government health care agencies are overseen by administrators, businessmen, and career politicians. In addition, private insurance companies and the pharmaceutical industry have significant influence over policy decisions that are not overseen by government public health agencies.

My wish for an ideal US health care system is one where the entire system would be overseen and managed by health care professionals, experts in public health, and health care economists. This leadership, as is the case with the Federal Reserve or NASA, would function semi-independently from the federal and state government and be free to develop policies based on science and cost-effectiveness. Health care resources would also be under the control of these independent groups of professionals who would make use of robust data to make evidence-based decisions on how to best apportion public funding of the health care system.

Reality Check

But how realistic are these wishes? Are they just some pie-in-the-sky dreams of an unachievable utopia, or are there any real-world precedents to which we can point?

It is unfortunate that there is no existing health care system that has all these attributes. There are some that have one or two, but none have all of them. But even if they did, it may not be enough to sell to the American people or to lawmakers. What we need is a precedent that has addressed the many uniquely American issues that will always come up with any prospective health care reform proposal.

One of the issues that has been a major hurdle in reform is the economic effects of health care policy. It is of such importance that it may be worth taking a closer look at how the health care and economic systems are related. It may also give us some ideas about how we can use this relationship to find a way to fix the current health care system.

CHAPTER 3

Health Care and the Economy

One thing that the COVID-19 pandemic has demonstrated beyond doubt is that a strong economy requires a healthy populace and a healthy health care system. But even before the pandemic, it was clear that the US health care system was closely intertwined with the economy. The concept of the "medical-industrial complex" was first proposed in the late 1960s and early 1970s. The term was meant to reflect the growing network of corporations that supply health care services and products for a profit, and was meant to be analogous to the military-industrial complex identified by President Eisenhower in the 1950s.

In 1980 the editor of the *New England Journal of Medicine* (NEJM), Arnold S. Relman, wrote:

> The most important health-care development of the day is the recent, relatively unheralded rise of a huge new industry that supplies health-care services for profit. Proprietary hospitals and nursing homes, diagnostic laboratories, homecare and emergency-room services, hemodialysis, and a wide variety of other services produced a gross income to this industry last year of about $35 billion to $40 billion.[1]

This medical-industrial complex has been very good for the US economy. By 2018 public health care spending accounted for 17.7% of the nation's gross domestic product, representing $11,172 per person.[2] This spending covered not only direct health care expenditures (like medical and pharmaceutical services) but also administrative services, which by 2018 represented more than 8% of the total. Hospital administration costs also rose and by 2011 (the most recent data available) reached 1.43% of gross domestic product ($667 per capita).[3]

So, who benefits from this substantial windfall to our economy?

It is not US *businesses* who benefit. Over the past 40 years, US businesses have become burdened with expenses that hamper profits, competition, and relations with their employees. Since the middle of the twentieth century, businesses have offered health insurance as a benefit to their employees. First it started as a fringe benefit, but soon it became an expected part of the benefit package. Then, under the ACA, it became a matter of federal law. In addition to the cost of insuring their employees, most of the larger businesses also have to select and manage the plans.

It is not US *employees* who benefit. For employees, the benefits of having health insurance are often offset by the high out-of-pocket costs. Employers manage their costs per employee, such that the money spent on health insurance premiums is not available for salary, meaning that effectively it is the employee who pays for their insurance through lost pay. In addition, many employees are stuck in a difficult dilemma: stay in a dead-end job or leave and lose their health insurance coverage. This dilemma is often exploited by employers who might feel less compelled to raise wages because they know that the employee needs the health insurance (and the employer needs to pay for it). And more generally, this dilemma also stifles employee mobility, something that is important in a modern economy. And many businesses may be reluctant to hire full-time employees because health insurance has become one of their fastest-growing costs.[4]

Early in the COVID-19 pandemic, 5.4 million people lost their health insurance in a matter of four months, because they were laid off.[5] Were it not for Medicaid being an option for some of the unemployed, the numbers of uninsured would have been much higher. Those states that had Medicaid expansion only saw 23% uninsured, while 43% of the unemployed workers in states that did not have Medicaid were also uninsured.

It is not US *consumers and patients* who benefit. Over the past four decades, the US health care consumer has seen a tremendous increase in the price for receiving health care. This can be seen in increases in out-of-pocket costs (premiums, deductibles, and co-payments) as well as from increased state and federal taxes.

One consumer group study found that total patient out-of-pocket spending reached an estimated $486 billion in 2016, having risen by 8% per year since 2011 from $250 per year in 1980 to over $1,400 in 2016 (an increase of over 45%, even after adjusting for inflation).[6] Workers are also spending 55% more on insurance premiums than a decade ago. Over the same time, their deductibles and co-pays are going up. Remarkably, on top of what people spend on health care through taxes and insurance, the average American now spends approximately $3,000 each year on services that are not covered. All this means that if you earn $52,000 a year, you are contributing $22,474, nearly half of your allocated wages, on health care.[7]

The health care consumer has also seen a growth in the limitation of access to health care providers and services. This limitation is not due to any medical concern but rather as a result of the economic pressures inherent in the current system. A good example of this is the insurance companies' practice of creating provider networks, sometimes called "Provider Panels." Health insurance carriers generally can define and adjust the number, the qualifications, and the quality of providers in their networks. They also may limit the number of providers in their networks as a means of conserving costs or coordinating care. In so doing, carriers may narrow their provider networks to an extent that enrollees in insurance plans may have extremely limited options when choosing providers.

Unfortunately, this practice of insurance companies often conflicts with the interests of providers, such as physicians, clinics, and hospitals, who seek the choice to treat patients needing their services, and the interests of patients, who often prefer, or medically need, a choice of providers, or the ability to use a particular provider.[8]

It is not US *doctors* who benefit. As significant as the changes over the past 20 years have been for businesses, employees, and consumers, the effects on health care providers have been stifling. Between the growth of bureaucratic hurdles from commercial insurance providers and unpredictable payment changes from Medicare and Medicaid, medical practices, hospitals, and other health care services have struggled to survive.

Physicians have been pushed to join large practices or health maintenance organizations that stress quantity of services over quality. These providers often have only minutes to see patients, and they have very little control over how their practices are run.

It has been pointed out by some that US physicians' fee-for-service charges are often twice those of their counterparts in other countries, and that this, in part, accounts for a major component of the higher per-capita cost of medical care in the US. These higher fees, it is argued, are brought about by robust lobbying efforts, through organizations like the American Medical Association and specialty groups. In many respects, the higher fees that US doctors charge are due to basic supply-demand pressures brought about by a lower number of physicians, per capita, than in most other industrialized countries (the US has approximately half the number of doctors per capita as Norway, Switzerland, or Germany).[9] It is also partly due to the higher proportion of doctors in medical specialties such as cardiology and neurosurgery, where salaries are substantially higher compared to salaries for primary care specialties such as internal medicine or pediatrics.

But it is also important to note that the need for lobbying efforts and higher fees are necessary reactions to pressures from working within the medical-industrial complex. In addition to the aforementioned higher administrative fees related to billing and credentialing, the US health care system has sufficiently more advanced technology than other countries. These beneficial technologies often require significantly higher levels of physician training and expertise to ensure the safety and effectiveness of the technology.

It is certainly true that many physicians do very well working within the medical-industrial complex, but these tend to be the exception rather than the rule. Most physicians make salaries equivalent to other professionals such as lawyers and engineers. In fact, physician incomes have generally gone down over the years, even as the length of required training to keep up with new knowledge and technologies, has gone up. Debt loads of newly minted doctors are huge, and are keeping some away from the profession, especially in primary care, which is increasingly being performed by advanced practice practitioners.

It *is* the *insurance and medical product* businesses that benefit. Insurance companies are the winners in the medical-industrial complex. About three-fifths of all Americans have employer-sponsored health insurance, yet there is surprisingly little oversight or uniformity of these plans. For the most part, these plans are negotiated with the individual businesses for coverage and price. Larger corporations have a greater say over both coverage and price, while smaller businesses must accept boiler-plate plans. Since these plans are largely opaque and use proprietary methods, businesses often have a difficult time comparing among them, often opting for the least expensive one without fully understanding the rules and limitations of coverage.

The insurance companies in turn use the enrolled employees as bargaining chips with hospitals and doctors to negotiate prices and services. Only those providers that agree to the terms are included in the panel of preferred providers. If a covered consumer wants to use an out-of-network provider, there is often a surcharge or no coverage at all.

The use of enrollees as bargaining chips effectively makes them assets (property) and the insurance companies that "own" them function as fiscal agents generating profits on the arbitrage as they pass money from the premium payer to the health care provider. This essentially makes insurance companies function like banks, where the assets are clients and patients instead of money or other forms of property. We will return to these bank-like roles of insurance companies in the next chapter.

The pharmaceutical and medical device industry in the United States has often been regarded as an entrepreneurial success story of innovation and quality. How much of this reputation is deserved is certainly questionable. Yet it has become an integral part of our economy and of the medical-industrial complex.

As drug and device prices have risen, therapies have become unaffordable for many people. To offset this, pharmaceutical companies negotiate special prices with commercial insurance companies, which increases insurance premiums and makes it more difficult for patients who lose insurance to get access to these therapies. In addition, public insurance plans like Medicare and Medicaid are not allowed to negotiate with the pharmaceutical and device companies, so HHS must either accept the set price or not offer the medicine (the consumer must then pay the full price out-of-pocket).

Even in its early stages, it was clear that the medical-industrial complex might be a significant impediment to health care delivery and a benefit to the insurance and pharmaceutical industry. In 1980 Dr. Relman of the *NEJM* recognized this trend:

> This new "medical–industrial complex" may be more efficient than its nonprofit competition, but it creates the problems of overuse and fragmentation of services, overemphasis on technology, and "cream-skimming," and it may also exercise undue influence on national health policy. In this medical market, physicians must act as discerning purchasing agents for their patients and therefore should have no conflicting financial interests. Closer attention from the public and the profession, and careful study, are necessary to ensure that the "medical–industrial-complex" puts the interests of the public before those of its stockholders.[1]

In the 40 years since this was written, the influence of for-profit health care organizations has only gotten stronger and more entrenched. Health insurance companies have slowly become health care management agencies and begun to regard their subscribers as assets (because "property" is too strong a word). These management agencies have their own set of providers (doctors and hospitals), their own set of rulemakers, and their own set of rules. They effectively became autonomous health care systems that compete with each other and with the publicly funded systems for subscribers and influence.

It would be remiss to ignore the insurance and pharmaceutical industries' prominence in the US economy. According to the US Bureau of Economic Analysis, insurance carriers and related activities contributed $564.5 billion, or 2.8%, to the nation's gross domestic product in 2018. The biopharmaceutical industry accounted for more than $1.2 trillion in economic output, representing 3.8% of total US output in 2014.

The commercial insurance industry, along with the pharmaceutical business, have thus become an integral part of the US economy. And, because of this, these two industries have had a tremendous amount of political influence that must be acknowledged when contemplating any reform initiatives.

The Medical-Industrial Complex and Health Care Reform

When one looks at the history of health care reform in the United States, it seems that the most successful attempts have been those that consider and address the existence of the medical-industrial complex. One of the key considerations is the inherent conflict between the "public" health care system, which is run by HHS, and the loose amalgamation of companies that makes up the "private" system. And it is important to understand that this private system is not just restricted to commercial *health insurance companies*, but includes the entire medical-industrial complex.

America's *public* health care system—which consists of the three health insurance programs (Medicare, Medicaid, and Indian Health Service), as well as several agencies, including the CDC, FDA, and NIH—is overseen by the Department of HHS, a cabinet-level agency that reports to the president and is funded by Congress. At the same time, the *private* system is quite disparate and uncoordinated, with autonomous health care management entities for which there is limited oversight, and which compete with each other and often, as we have seen, with the public system.

This inherent tension between HHS and the medical-industrial complex can be seen in the current landscape of health care reform. On one side, the "single payer" proponents want to completely eliminate (or at least significantly restrict) the medical-industrial complex and empower HHS to run all health insurance. On the other side the "free market" proponents would eliminate all public insurance (like Medicare and Medicaid) and let the private sector run the insurance market (like automobile insurance).

The ACA was an attempted compromise between these extremes that ended up upsetting both camps. The free-market proponents didn't like it because it expanded public insurance (mostly through Medicaid) and imposed an individual mandate that required everyone to have some kind of health insurance. The single-payer proponents did not like the huge payments to commercial insurance that they considered handouts. And neither camp was happy, but for different reasons, with the ACA's business mandate requiring businesses with more than 50 workers to offer health insurance to their employees.

Supporters of the ACA point out that the legislation did expand health insurance coverage for 20 million people and that there was an attempt to make insurance more affordable. They believe that strengthening some aspects of the HIMs to increase competition (with a public option) and making other modifications will fix the issues the ACA is facing. However, almost everyone agrees that the ACA is no more than a stopgap measure until we can get a better plan.

So, what is the solution?

One answer might lie in studying the history of American banking and financial reform in the early years of the twentieth century.

CHAPTER 4

Lessons from the Creation of the Federal Reserve System

Historical Parallels

Prior to the establishment of the Federal Reserve (the Fed) in 1913, the US banking and financial system was in turmoil, suffering from many of the issues currently facing the health care system. Problems such as a lack of infrastructure, a lack of oversight, and too many political and financial influences, created a chaotic banking and monetary system.[1] The formation of the Fed as a semi-independent agency, run by economists and guided by tested economic principles, brought much-needed order to the banking system, and modernized the US economy.

It is remarkable how the current debates over health care reform have many parallels to those when the banking reforms were required that led to the creation of the Fed. For example, arguments for and against a single-payer system (or Medicare for All) overseen by HHS are similar to the arguments over 100 years ago for and against having a "central bank" overseen by the Department of the Treasury (also a cabinet-level agency answering to the president). In the alternative, those who wanted independent banks with little federal oversight would probably also advocate today for strengthening the role of private insurance at the expense of the public system. And the arguments for and against maintaining and fixing the ACA parallel the arguments for and against keeping the system created under the National Bank Act of 1863, which allowed banks significant autonomy with a decentralized currency.

The result of the decades-long debate over these choices for banking reform was a fourth choice: the Federal Reserve Act of 1913, which created a relatively independent Federal Reserve board of governors with a well-defined infrastructure that was equipped with the modern economic tools to manage the US banking and monetary system. For those advocating a central bank, there was a unified banking and monetary system under the Federal Reserve Bank. For those advocating for stronger banks, the act gave them economic stability and a seat at the table. And the Federal Reserve's independence allowed for less political and financial influence over its decisions and actions.

How this system stabilized the economic and financial health of the United States is beyond the purview of this book, but there is no doubt that its oversight and expert management was instrumental in helping the US become the world's leading economic and financial force.

Would a Fed-like structure help the health care system the same way the Fed helped the banking system? To answer this question let's take a closer look at the history of US health care reform.

Since the enactment of Medicare in 1965 (the first and most successful attempt at reform), Congress's role in health care has gradually increased. This is because Congress is responsible for financing public programs like Medicare and Medicaid. At first their role was purely financial, but as Medicare and Medicaid spending began to increase, Congress became interested in ways to curb the cost. Over the years, Congress made several attempts to hold down Medicare spending. One instructive example was an effort called the sustainable growth rate (SGR). The SGR attempted to address an inherent incentive in the US health care system for doctors and hospitals to do more procedures and to avoid (or at least ignore) prevention. It did this by tying Medicare Part B payments (to physicians and other providers) to US GDP. Its goal was to ensure that the yearly increase in the expense per Medicare beneficiary did not exceed the growth in GDP. If Medicare expenditures for the previous year exceeded the target expenditures, then the conversion factor would decrease payments to physicians for the next year. If the expenditures were less than expected, the conversion factor would increase the payments.

Right from the start, the SGR was a failure. It quickly became evident that physicians had only modest control over Medicare spending and the gap between GDP and Medicare spending grew quickly. Most of the increases were attributed to increases in pharmaceutical and device costs. More importantly, if Congress went through with the prescribed cut in Medicare payments to physicians, physicians might not be able to afford to take Medicare patients. This would in turn significantly limit Medicare patients (who were also voters) from accessing medical care. For this reason, every year Congress suspended or adjusted the cuts (this was referred to as a "doc fix"), thereby regularly and effectively "kicking the can down the road." But each time it was postponed, the gap grew so that by the time the SGR was replaced in 2015 (see below) the potential pay cut to physicians was close to 25%.

Congress then took another approach, called the Medicare Access and CHIP Reauthorization Act (MACRA), also known as the "permanent doc fix." For decades most professional medical societies in the United States have been publishing science-based clinical guidelines that emphasize the need to promote preventive services. These guidelines also emphasize that some more expensive procedures are no more effective (and sometimes less effective) than less aggressive approaches. They recognized that the current system had inherent financial incentives to spend more time on procedures and the treatment of diseases and less incentive for preventative efforts. In MACRA, Congress attempted to change this dynamic by linking Medicare payments to doctors based on "quality" rather than quantity.

However, Congress chose quality without either defining what it means or explaining how to measure it. Instead, it left it up to the HHS and physician groups to set up experimental programs—programs that relied more on economic incentives than actual outcomes. These "payment models"—with names such as MIPs (merit-based incentive payment system), APMs (alternative payment models), and ACOs (accountable care organizations)—primarily incentivize cutting costs by profit-sharing rather than directly promoting evidence-based outcomes. The reason for this is that in the current health care system infrastructure, it is much easier for Congress and HHS to modify health care delivery through cost reduction incentive models rather than through programs that promote evidence-based practice.

Finally, there was the Affordable Care Act. According to the Kaiser Family Foundation, the ACA reduced the number of uninsured nonelderly Americans by 20 million, dropping to a historic low in 2016.[2] From 2010, when the ACA was introduced, the uninsured fell from 47 million to 27 million in 2016 (a more than 40% fall). However, the insurance that these formerly uninsured received was not all the same. Many received their new insurance from the Healthcare.gov marketplace, but almost 75% of the newly insured were through Medicaid.

There are several things that need to be understood about Medicaid, especially when it comes to the ACA. Because it is a program that is supported by both the federal government and individual state governments, there was a significant variation in how well funded the Medicaid program was in each state. Some states fully funded the program, allowing full participation. Other states refused to fund the program, resulting in a much weaker program. In addition, many providers did not want to take Medicaid because of the historically lower reimbursement rates. The ACA attempted to fix this by raising reimbursement to Medicare levels, but the reputation of Medicaid could not be overcome.

The overall result of the ACA is that it did significantly raise the number of people who have insurance, but it did little to raise the quality of the insurance or the access that people with insurance have to health care providers.

This all invites the question: Why has it been so hard for Congress to create legislation that can achieve the changes that would make the system more effective and more efficient?

One reason is that Congress, like HHS, only has oversight over the part of the health care system that is publicly funded, and so it is limited to reforming Medicare, Medicaid, and Indian Health Service. The lack of any significant congressional oversight over commercial insurance makes any health care legislation significantly less effective. Although commercial insurers might eventually adopt changes made to Medicare or Medicaid, doing so is usually voluntary and implemented on a case-by-case and insurer-by-insurer basis. This may result in different policies depending on the insurance carrier, causing a heterogeneous mosaic of coverage and policy with no clear master plan, creating an inefficiency of chaos.

The parallels between the banking and financial turmoil of the early twentieth century and the dysfunctional health care system of the twenty-first century consist of three overarching problems found in each of these complex situations: conflicting interests, a lack of a unified organizational infrastructure, and the lack of a single independent (and nonpartisan) oversight body with the authority to control the entire system.

As many commercial insurance organizations have undertaken roles and functions in the health care system that are like those of banks in our financial system, why not create a similar structure for our health care system as was created over a hundred years ago for our banking system? Why not form an independent agency (or board) and create a modern unified infrastructure for it to oversee?

Following the lessons learned during the creation of the Federal Reserve System, Congress could legislate the creation of a "National Medical Board." This NMB could be organized in a way very similar to the Federal Reserve System, with a chair, a board of governors, and an advisory council. The chair would be required to have specific credentials that would make them suited for the job. At the minimum, they would need to be a physician with experience and training in public health, health care administration, and health care economics.

The board of governors would represent various aspects of the health care system, such as patients, hospitals, physicians, nursing, insurance (public and private), the non-business aspects of pharmaceuticals and devices, research, and communications (and others).

To help insulate the board of governors from special interests, a separate advisory board would be established. Made up of representatives of the many medical-industrial complex special interests such as businesses, the business side of the pharmaceutical industry, and commercial insurance companies, this board would help the governors and its chair understand how its policies might affect these interests.

Much like the Federal Reserve, the NMB would be independent of the executive branch of the federal government, giving it a much-needed autonomy to create policies based on science, with a minimum of political pressure. It would also be more insulated from the influence of the medical-industrial complex special interests but would still recognize the important role these concerns play in the economy and would take into account their interests in an open and transparent way.

CHAPTER 5

How a National Medical Board Can Help the Current Health Care System's Problems

Out of intense complexities, intense simplicities emerge.
—Winston Churchill, *The World Crisis*

The complexity of the US health care system is almost unfathomable. This is true whether we are considering the complexity of insurance, infrastructure, research, or politics. And it is the reason why health care reform is so difficult. Paradoxically, it seems that the simple solution is to completely scrap the current system and build a new one from the ground up. But this is a very scary proposition.

It is scary because many people are understandably afraid of change. This fear is not necessarily the fear of losing what they have but rather not knowing how the change might affect them and, more importantly, if it would actually work. For this reason, any attempt at health care reform in the US needs a plan that is based on tried-and-true methods, not methods that work in other countries, but ones that have been tested in the US.

Luckily, we have a great precedent when it comes to restructuring and simplifying our health care system. The Federal Reserve System was created specifically to fit the US ethos of independence, entrepreneurial spirit, and a healthy distrust of the federal government. The Federal Reserve was not the typical central bank found in most European countries. This enabled it to remain somewhat insulated from both political and special interest pressures.

How would a Fed-like National Medical Board be the starting point to solving the US health care crisis? It would consolidate and unify the entire health care system under one body, reduce political and financial influence, be more trusted, and be relatively easy to create through legislation.

Consolidation and Unification

The NMB would take all of the many elements of the current health care system and put them under one roof. Currently, no single agency performs this function, and many of the agencies or groups that do exist have overlapping jurisdictions and rarely cooperate. Government agencies—such as HHS and VHA—and the unregulated private insurance industry, make up a complex and inefficient mosaic of health care oversight and services, with no clear master plan.

Agencies that currently oversee the public portion of the health care system within HHS, would become governorships in the board of governors. For example, oversight of the CDC would be moved to a Governor of Disease Control and Prevention, oversight of the FDA would be moved to a Governor of Diagnostics, Therapeutics and Nutrition, and oversight of the NIH and Agency for Healthcare Research and Quality (AHRQ) would be moved to a Governor of Health Care Research (the ultimate makeup and titles of these governorships might be different). In addition, the public health benefit plans—Medicare, Medicaid, Indian Health Service, and the VHA—as well as all commercial insurance plans would be consolidated under a Governor for Health Care Benefits. This would allow for well-defined oversight as well as facilitate the establishment of a more comprehensive, efficient, effective, and equitable benefits system (discussed in the next chapter). The NMB board of governors would also oversee other aspects of the health care system often overlooked. It would oversee all medical data from all providers (discussed in the next chapter), and the credentialing of hospitals, nursing homes, doctors, nurses, and other medical personnel.

This comprehensive oversight of all aspects of the health care system would create a truly unified system, with maximal efficiency and minimal duplication. It would also consolidate government agencies and remove benefit determinations from other government agencies and commercial interests.

Independence and Reduction of Political and Financial Influence

It is unlikely that any proposed plan could completely remove financial or political influences altogether. However, the relative independence of a Fed-like NMB would set up a significant buffer to such influences, much like the Federal Reserve System did for its oversight of the economy.

According to the Federal Reserve's website:

> Congress has determined the Federal Reserve can best achieve its mission of supporting maximum employment and stable prices as an independent agency that makes decisions based on the best available evidence and analysis, without taking politics into consideration.
>
> Experience around the world has also shown that countries with independent central banks that are able to make decisions free from political influence have better economic outcomes for their citizens.[1]

For the same reasons, this independence would also be important for an effective health care system. However, the mission would be different. Instead of "supporting maximum employment and stable prices" the NMB's mission would be "To promote the health of each and every person in the United States of America."

Trust

An inherent distrust of the federal government is as old as the United States itself. This distrust has never been as evident as when it comes to health care policy. The thought of having some lawmaker or bureaucrat being in charge of health benefits has been anathema since Medicare was first proposed. In 1961 Ronald Reagan made a major political impact with his recording of *Ronald Reagan Speaks Out Against Socialized Medicine*, in which he said, "We can say right now that we want no further encroachment on these individual liberties and freedoms. And at the moment, the key issue is we do not want socialized medicine."[2] This mistrust of the federal government is not limited to those on the Right. During the COVID-19 pandemic, many on the Left decried the Trump administration's Coronavirus Task Force for overruling recommendations from the CDC and infectious disease specialists such as Dr. Anthony Fauci.

The issue of trust, or mistrust, is not limited to the federal government. There is an equal wariness of the commercial insurance industry. The distrust is much deeper than just not trusting what they are selling. It is also the mistrust of what these companies do with the personal data they collect. In 2018 Pro Publica reported:

> At a time when every week brings a new privacy scandal and worries abound about the misuse of personal information, patient advocates and privacy scholars say the insurance industry's data gathering runs counter to its touted, and federally required, allegiance to patients' medical privacy.[3]

The insurance industry asserts that these data are used to improve patient health, but in a for-profit and generally unregulated industry that uses its clients as bargaining chips with providers, other uses cannot be ruled out.

Because the NMB would be neither a part of the federal government nor commercial insurance, it should be significantly more trusted to handle patient data.

Easy to Legislate

Possibly the biggest advantage of modeling the NMB after the Federal Reserve is that it makes drafting health care reform legislation easier. The challenge of legislating for health care reform comes from the inherent problem that Congress only has limited jurisdiction over the system. The Constitution does give Congress the power to make laws regarding interstate commerce, which is the reason most reform has been limited to matters that could be considered interstate commerce, for example, insurance coverage. This was true with Medicare, for which a trust fund was established, for the sustainable growth rate legislation, and for the ACA. What Congress cannot legislate is how to practice medicine. Yet, many of the laws that Congress has enacted have had major unintended consequences, precisely because the laws only deal with insurance aspects of medical practice.

By establishing and funding a NMB, Congress could get out of the business of legislating health care policy and back to its core role: financial and fiduciary oversight. It would be the NMB board that would be responsible for figuring out how to allocate the funding across all aspects of the health care system, whether for public health, hospitals, research, or informatics.

As will be seen in subsequent chapters, Congress would also need to give the NMB certain permissions, including the ability to pay providers, bill patients, and collect from insurance companies. It would also have to assign the NMB authority to regulate interstate commerce in health care.

How would all this work out? How would the NMB be able to succeed where all other attempts have failed? It starts with the understanding that to be effective in the twenty-first century, any reform plan must have a holistic approach to reforming the *entire infrastructure* of the US health care system and not just insurance. Congress must give the NMB the tools to be able to use all modern technologies most effectively to enable it to accomplish this lofty goal.

CHAPTER 6

EMBRACE

A Comprehensive Plan for Health Care System Reform

You can't solve a problem on the same level that it was created. You have to rise above it to the next level.
—attributed to Albert Einstein

When one thinks of all the health care reform efforts that have been proposed in the past 60 years, it is easy to forget that almost all have been limited to reforming health insurance. Whether it is creating public insurance with Medicare and Medicaid, or expanding private insurance with the ACA, there was little effort to reform health care infrastructure or quality. The few attempts to improve quality, as in MACRA, have been generally ineffective and have had the regularly observed side effects of increased complexity and administrative burden to providers.

It is remarkable that all these proposals, at least the ones that are given any attention by lawmakers, were crafted by political think tanks or corporations deeply entrenched in the medical-industrial complex, rather than by health care professionals. This is a lost opportunity, since a solution to the problems of the US health care system would benefit from input from those who work within it every day, who know both its strengths and weaknesses, and who have direct connections with the patients who use it. Health care professionals understand that attempting to reform health care delivery simply by increasing the number of insured Americans or changing the way doctors and hospitals are reimbursed, often have unintended consequences such as increasing bureaucratic burdens or creating misdirected incentives in patient care.

EMBRACE (**E**xpanding **M**edical and **B**ehavioral **R**esources with **A**ccess to **C**are for **E**veryone) is unique among health care reform proposals for three reasons. First, it is the only proposal for a complete overhaul of the health system infrastructure, not just health insurance. Second, it is the only proposal to be created by health care professionals. And third, it is the only plan that will give health care professionals the command and the tools to run the health care system with relative insulation from government and commercial pressures.

It was constructed over many years by a group of doctors, nurses, public health experts, and health care economists who felt that a new approach was needed. An approach that would be focused on patient health and outcomes rather than insurance and cost. One that would create an infrastructure that could deliver evidence-based modern care with minimal administrative or financial burdens. An approach that would create a health care system that puts health care over politics or financial pressures.

EMBRACE was born out of the experience of misaligned bureaucratic burdens and unintended consequences that clinicians encountered every day in the US health care system, and a wish to be free of the increasingly acrimonious political discourse that surrounds health care policy.

From when it was first proposed, the group recognized that to be truly effective and efficient, any plan for reform needed to include a comprehensive change to the infrastructure of the system. It needed to allow for all the new innovations in medicine and in communications. And it needed to bring order to the chaotic mosaic of agencies and insurance schemes that made up the US health care system.

The group considered many of the existing proposals, to see if they would meet these needs. They first asked, "Why not adopt a 'single-payer system' in the United States, or expand Medicare to cover the entire population (and eliminate private insurance)?" The first issue with single-payer and Medicare for All options is that they only deal with insurance reform and do little to change the system's archaic infrastructure. In addition, neither option is politically or economically viable in a country where private insurance accounted for 30% of national health expenditures and almost 6% of the GDP in 2012.[1] Even if Congress had the political will to go against the very powerful insurance lobby, it would be hard pressed to find a model in any Western country that did not have some form of private insurance available to its population. Even systems in countries that single-payer advocates hold up as possible models for the United States to follow, have developed a rather robust private insurance sector. These private payers often compete with the public system for the healthier and less "needy" patients, leaving the public sector with a patient population that is sicker and costs more to treat. And this increased cost usually leads to fewer resources and poorer service in the public system. This could even lead to a bipartite health care system, with an efficient, full-featured private system for those who can afford it and a slow, inefficient, and expensive public system for the majority of the population.

Importantly, the single-payer models that have fared best in this conflict between commercial and public insurance have been those that have made an attempt at integration in a way that reduces the competition for patients between the two. This, in essence, is how the EMBRACE proposal is organized: a "public" system that covers the basic health care needs of the entire population, but allows private insurance to cover what the "public" system does not cover.

But, instead of organizing this system as an afterthought or as a fix of a single-payer model, EMBRACE incorporates both public and private sectors as one seamless system. It still offers many incentives for the private insurers (and their stockholders), yet it would most likely make it significantly less expensive for consumers to purchase private insurance and easier for them to understand what they are getting, than in our current system.

EMBRACE is constructed to modernize health care in a way that would bring the US system into the twenty-first century, while maintaining most of the best aspects of the existing system. It would be user-friendly and would significantly reduce consumer concerns such as bankruptcy or lack of coverage. But probably the most important thing that EMBRACE would bring, is a health care system that is *designed* to deliver the best health care to the entire US population, something that cannot be said about the current system, or any other proposal being considered.

What follows is an attempt to outline the current state of the proposal. It is by no means sacrosanct. Indeed, since it was first proposed in 2009,[2] it has undergone several updates that reflect feedback from various sources, and will no doubt benefit from further improvements.

EMBRACE is founded on three principal innovations that are designed to work together: an evidence-based three-tiered benefits (insurance) system; a web-based, nationwide Healthcare Information Platform; and an independent National Medical Board that would oversee the entire health care system. Collectively this would create a unified health care system with universal coverage.

The Tiered Benefits System

The evidence-based tiered benefits system, a main pillar of EMBRACE's infrastructure, consists of three levels:

- Tier 1 (the basic level) applies to all conditions that have been determined to be life threatening, all services that have been shown to be life extending, and all therapies that have been shown to prevent life-threatening conditions.
- Tier 2 applies to all conditions that have been shown to affect quality of life, therapies that have been shown to improve these conditions, and services and therapies for Tier 1 conditions that lack the scientific evidence to be included under Tier 1 coverage.
- Tier 3 applies to "luxury" services as well as conditions not covered in Tiers 1 and 2.

The determination of the conditions and therapies covered by each of the tiers would ultimately be made by the NMB, the nongovernmental agency modeled after the Federal Reserve, and would be predominantly based on scientific studies and published medical guidelines. Consequently, it is difficult to predict all the conditions that might be included in each of the tiers. However, based on some of the current published evidence and guidelines, some reasonable conjectures can be made.

Tier 1. Examples of conditions covered under Tier 1 would most likely include acute myocardial infarctions (heart attacks), cancer, pregnancy, and severe depression. This tier would also likely include treatment of conditions that have been shown to increase the risk of developing life-threatening illnesses, such as hypertension, diabetes, and hyperlipidemia. In addition, this tier covers all testing used to rule in or rule out a Tier 1 condition. For example: if a patient presents to the emergency room with chest pains, Tier 1 covers any of the scientifically validated tests performed in the workup until a Tier 1 condition (such as a myocardial infarction) is diagnosed or definitively excluded. Any other testing would fall under Tier 2.

Tier 2. Conditions covered by Tier 2 include those that may significantly affect quality of life but that have not been shown to affect life expectancy or increase the risk of other life-threatening conditions. These might include osteoarthritis, low back pain, plaque psoriasis, and irritable bowel syndrome. In addition, this tier covers therapies for life-threatening conditions and workups that still require scientific proof of efficacy in order to be covered in Tier 1.

Tier 3. This tier is reserved for "luxury" treatments and procedures that have little or no scientific evidence of reducing mortality or improving quality of life, such as facelifts and LASIK surgery.

The main reason for creating benefit tiers is to determine coverage. EMBRACE, unlike single-payer systems, would allow both public and private insurers to participate, but defines services to be covered by payer type. Because Tier 1 conditions are the most serious in terms of both personal and public health, they would be covered by a form of public insurance. This coverage would be automatic and universal and not dependent on age, gender, employment status, preexisting conditions, or even military service. It would cover the entire population from cradle to grave.

Tier 2 would be paid out-of-pocket or covered by commercial insurance. Consumers who want Tier 2 coverage could purchase it through a computer-based program modeled after the successful Medigap menu of plans. Medigap (private health insurance plans sold as a supplement to traditional Medicare) has been working well since its introduction in the early 1990s. Its menu allows the consumer to easily compare the features of the various plans available. Table 6.1 is an example of the Medigap menu.

The rows in Table 6.1 represent specific features contained in the various insurance plans listed in the columns. For example, if you want a comprehensive program that covers each benefit row, you might choose plan F, while plan A offers bare-bones coverage. Once consumers have chosen the plan that best suits their needs, they can check, on a linked menu, which insurance companies offer the plan and the range of premiums. No other method of purchasing private health insurance in the United States allows the consumer to compare features and prices of commercial insurance as well as Medigap.

EMBRACE would offer a similar menu of private insurance offerings for those consumers who want to add on to their automatic Tier 1 coverage. Instead of the supplements to Medicare insurance, this menu would list features of Tier 2 coverage plans. The ability to compare these policies side by side would allow consumers to first find the best Tier 2 plan for their needs and then to find the best price. As with Medigap, consumers would be able to shop for plans online and verify the minimal standards of the Tier 2 plan they select.

This menu of plans would be accessible through a computerized marketplace called the HealthMart (this is the name the group chose, but it could be changed). HealthMart would be modeled after Medigap rather than the HIM that is offered under the ACA.

Through the HealthMart, Tier 2 plans may be very general, or they may be very specific for particular groups, such as the elderly, veterans, or factory workers. They may be offered through supplements by the federal government (as a substitute for Medicare), VA (as a substitute for veteran benefits), or employers (for disability insurance, worker's compensation not covered by Tier 1, or as a limited bonus).

Because Tier 1 covers most catastrophic medical occurrences, such

Table 6.1 Comparison of Medigap Plans

Medigap benefits	Medigap plans									
	A	B	C	D	F	G	K	L	M	N
Part A coinsurance and hospital costs up to an additional 365 days after Medicare benefits are depleted	Yes	Yes	Yes	Yes	Yes	Yes	Yes	Yes	Yes	Yes
Part B co-insurance or co-payment	Yes	Yes	Yes	Yes	Yes	Yes	50%	75%	Yes	Yes
Blood (first three pints)	Yes	Yes	Yes	Yes	Yes	Yes	50%	75%	Yes	Yes
Part A hospice care co-insurance or co-payment	Yes	Yes	Yes	Yes	Yes	Yes	50%	75%	Yes	Yes
Skilled nursing facility care co-insurance	No	No	Yes	Yes	Yes	Yes	50%	75%	Yes	Yes
Part A deductible	No	Yes	Yes	Yes	Yes	Yes	50%	75%	50%	Yes
Part B deductible	No	No	Yes	No	Yes	No	No	No	No	No
Part B excess charges	No	No	No	No	Yes	Yes	No	No	No	No
Foreign travel exchange (up to plan limits)	No	No	Yes	Yes	Yes	Yes	No	No	Yes	Yes
Out-of-pocket limit	N/A	N/A	N/A	N/A	N/A	N/A	$4,940	$2,470	N/A	N/A

Note: Yes = plan meets 100% of benefits. No = plan does not cover that benefit. Percentage (%) = plan covers the noted percentage of the benefit. N/A = benefit is not applicable for that plan.

as trauma or cancer, it is likely that the price of the optional Tier 2 coverage would be significantly lower than that of current health insurance policies. This means that most Tier 2 plans should be affordable for the average consumer. In addition, unlike current commercial policies offered through a job or a HIM (either state run or federally managed plans under the ACA), any policy purchased under EMBRACE would be fully portable throughout the United States.

Tier 2 plans would also be available through other means. They could be offered as hiring incentives, veteran benefits, rewards for meeting certain preventive goals (in Tier 1), such as quitting smoking or losing a certain amount of weight, or even as an age-based substitute for Medicare.

Unlike the current system, there would be no need to provide proof of insurance for a doctor's visit or scheduled procedure. Instead, all insurance information would be computerized and immediately available to the health care provider.

Finally, on average, the overall health-care related cost to consumers under EMBRACE would be equal to or less than what they currently pay. Today, most consumers pay for health care in many different ways—so many that it is difficult to know the true cost. There are premium payments (that are often hidden in payroll deductions for employer-provided insurance), payroll deductions meant to support the Medicare Trust Fund, and several forms of out-of-pocket payments, such as deductibles and co-payments. Some insurance policies offer different coverage depending on the contracted provider network, charging a penalty if the consumer goes out-of-network, and premiums can change if the consumer moves or changes jobs.

Tier 3 services would generally not be covered by insurance, which is typical of the current system.

The Healthcare Information Platform

Although the services in the three tiers are covered by different payers, they would all be connected by a centralized platform called the Healthcare Information Platform (HIP). The HIP would be a secure web-based system available to every licensed health care provider. On the provider side (doctor, nurse, physical therapist, hospital, nursing home, etc.), a single patient encounter page—the Universal Billing Form (UBF)—would apply to all patient encounters. The provider completes this form and submits it electronically to a central computer with the completed electronic patient chart. This central computer would analyze the data and determine to which tier the patient's condition and services correspond. If a Tier 1 service is determined, the provider is paid immediately. A Tier 2 determination leads to an automated computerized search for insurance and, if private insurance coverage exists, the insurance company is notified. If the patient has no insurance for a service determined to fall under a Tier 2 or Tier 3 plan, the HIP bills the patient for the service on behalf of the provider. (All Tier 1 services are covered, regardless of the patient's insurance status.)

The UBF addresses the inefficiency of the current billing system. Over the years, the bureaucracy that has built up around insurance billing has become one of the most burdensome and wasteful aspects of medical practice. Medical providers must either spend hours dealing with forms and discussing cases with insurance companies or hire others to do so. Patients are also increasingly caught in this process. In addition, insurance companies spend a lot of time and money to screen these claims. Under the current system, this screening process is an essential component of the companies' business models but significantly increases cost. Because EMBRACE virtually eliminates these burdensome and wasteful hurdles, it has been estimated that a system that can streamline the process can save as much as $350 billion annually.[3]

Beyond the HIP's billing functions, access to its web-based platform would be available to application developers. Similar to the manner in which the Apple platform supports Apple devices, such as the iPhone and iPad, while allowing entrepreneurs to develop millions of apps, the HIP would be available to developers for application development that could be used by the entire health care system. Applications such as electronic medical records would be especially welcome, as many of those currently offered have the disadvantage of not being interoperable. This inability to freely exchange information electronically among the various electronic medical records increases health care costs and adversely affects patient care.

The common platform and the stipulation that all patient data be easily accessible to providers not only would make the EMBRACE system more efficient but also provide an opportunity to obtain direct data on almost all aspects of medical care. Currently, data collection is inefficient, costly, and relatively unreliable, which makes the routine monitoring of health care quality difficult. As part of the EMBRACE infrastructure, the HIP would allow for real-time feedback on public health programs, drug and device efficacy and safety, and even the early detection of developing epidemics. Additionally, the HIP would be a platform for undertaking health care research in the real world of patient care. This would have been particularly helpful during the COVID-19 pandemic for tracking the spread of the virus and for rapid development of diagnostics and effective therapies.

The National Medical Board

Data analysis and the subsequent ability to act are difficult without a centralized agency to oversee all aspects of the nation's very large and complex health care system. Under EMBRACE, all aspects of the current complex and inefficient mosaic of health care oversight and services would be unified and streamlined under the NMB.

EMBRACE proposes the creation of an independent oversight body based on the Federal Reserve System to oversee the entire American health care system. I am calling this body the NMB, but other names might be considered, such as Universal Healthcare Board, or Unified Healthcare Board. The ultimate structure of the NMB will largely depend on Congress, but using the Federal Reserve as a model, it might look something like that shown in Figure 6.1.

The chair of the NMB, a physician with experience in public health and health care economics, would be appointed by the president and confirmed by the Senate for a 5- or 10-year term. As with the Federal Reserve System, there would be a board of governors that would have representation of all parts of the health care system. This would in-

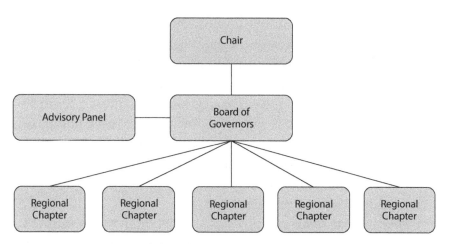

FIGURE 6.1. Organizational chart showing the relationships of the various components of the NMB. The chair would have direct oversight of the board of governors, which in turn would have oversight of the various regional chapters. An advisory panel would represent commercial and advocacy groups associated with health care.

clude governors overseeing public health (replacing the CDC), drugs and devices (replacing the FDA), health care system research (replacing the NIH, AHRQ), tier system administration (which would include public benefits, private benefits, and guideline development), patient-centered care, nursing, hospitals, veterans' health care administration (replacing the VHA), HIP administration, medical imaging, medical laboratory administration, post-graduate medical education, and others as needed.

An advisory panel would represent special commercial groups, such as the pharmaceutical industry, device companies, private insurance firms, and businesses, and various advocacy groups representing patient, physician, hospital, and religious concerns. The advisory panel would have a special relationship with the board. As the group represents the special interest groups that make up the medical-industrial complex and other vital special interest groups, it is important that they be represented in the deliberations of the board.

The board would determine the specifics of its relationship with this panel and how it would be organized. But it is likely that there would be a concerted effort to separate the science from the business and political aspect as much as possible. For example, it is likely that there would be a governor for therapeutics with representation from pharmaceutical and device companies that would be strictly represented by the science-based side of these corporations. At the same time, the business aspect of pharmaceutical and device firms will be represented in the advisory panel. There may also be separation of the advocacy side of groups representing patients (such as the American Association of Retired Persons), doctors (American Medical Association), and hospitals into the advisory panel and the science side of the same groups that work with the board.

Since there is significant geographic variation in health care, the NMB would have regional chapters. these regional chapters would survey their region for health trends such as epidemics or drug abuse, and be better able to respond with region-specific solutions.

The NMB will have many functions, with its top priority being the oversight of the tiered benefits system and the determination of the tier assignments of all conditions and services. Initially, these tier assignments will be determined by using all available scientific evidence of testing algorithms, illness severity, and treatment effectiveness. Of course, most of the studies currently available are not designed with the intention of advancing health care delivery in general and EMBRACE specifically. Therefore, the NMB would eventually need to commission its own studies.

Pharmaceutical and medical device companies design and finance most of the large studies on therapy in order to obtain product approval. Consequently, the resulting information is difficult to apply to actual clinical use. Moreover, objective comparative outcome data (i.e., information on how particular drugs or devices perform against others) is virtually nonexistent. In addition, these studies often enroll limited types of patients (e.g., only patients over the age of sixty-five), so the resultant data are also limited in their clinical usefulness.

Under EMBRACE, the NMB would be able to commission studies designed to facilitate tier assignment specifically and ensure that the research has maximal effect on public health. As these studies are completed, the NMB would be able to fine-tune the various tier assignments.

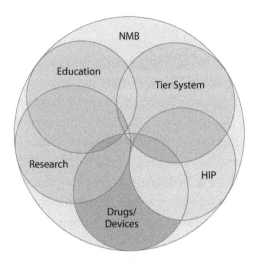

FIGURE 6.2. The EMBRACE "unified" health care system

A *Unified* Health Care System

Together, these three innovations would form a unified health care system integrating twenty-first century technology and infrastructure overseen by the NMB. As represented in Figure 6.2, the NMB would have control over the entire US health care system through its governorships, including the tier system of public and private insurance benefits, the HIP, drugs and devices, medical research, and post-graduate education of all health care professionals.

Although the governorships would be separate departments, there would likely be significant overlap for many of their interests and jurisdictions. However, because they are unified under one chair and a common mission ("To promote the health of each and every person in the United States of America"), it is likely that many of the barriers to cooperation that now exist would be alleviated in this new system.

Precedents

As drastic as these changes might seem at first blush, many of the elements of the EMBRACE proposal have precedents in the United States.

Precedents for the Tier System

A method very close to the tiered benefits system of organizing benefits (insurance) coverage already exists in "original" or "traditional" Medicare. What is not covered by the basic Medicare plans can be supplemented by a Medigap plan. The Medigap program was started in 1990 and offers supplemental private insurance for original Medicare recipients to cover what has been termed the "donut hole" in Medicare coverage, such as the 20% deductible fees on outpatient and hospital observation care, co-payments, and other uncovered services. This method of separation of coverage is very similar to how the EMBRACE tiered benefits system is organized. Table 6.2 compares how the different tiers correlate to the various types of Medicare coverage.

Publicly covered Tier 1 benefits under EMBRACE correspond to Medicare Parts A and B that are funded by the Medicare trust funds. Tier 2, which would be covered by commercial insurance under EMBRACE, is very similar to the Medigap system that provides supplemental coverage for what basic Medicare does not cover and would otherwise be paid out-of-pocket by the patient. In fact, Medigap was the inspiration for the EMBRACE Tier 2 menu of plans, as well as for the feasibility of having private insurance participate in a public benefits program.

The ultimate distribution of coverage between Tier 1 and Tier 2 under EMBRACE would likely be very different from that under Medicare and Medigap. Instead of the rather arbitrary services and fees that are left uncovered under Medicare Parts A and B and picked up by Medigap, EMBRACE will divide the coverage between Tier 1 and Tier 2 using evidence-based data to prioritize lifesaving, life-sustaining, and preventive services.

Tier 3 has no corresponding category for Medicare recipients, meaning that these luxury services are usually paid out-of-pocket, just as proposed for EMBRACE.

As is true with EMBRACE Tier 1, Medicare is publicly financed and, as with Tier 2, Medigap is offered by commercial insurance providers through a menu of plans. The choices on the Medigap menu are deter-

Table 6.2 EMBRACE Compared with "Traditional Medicare"

EMBRACE	Medicare
Tier 1	Part A and Part B
Tier 2	Medigap
Tier 3	Not Addressed

mined by the Centers for Medicare & Medicaid Services (CMS) and the insurance companies have the choice of whether to offer the particular supplemental plan. However, if the commercial insurance provider agrees to offer a particular plan, it must make the plan available in all states. Medigap plan prices are allowed to vary from state to state because health care in some areas is more expensive than in other areas. Private insurance plans purchased through Medigap also offer better access to physicians and hospitals, because they must follow the same rules as traditional Medicare. These same rules would also be true with the EMBRACE tier system.

Precedents for the Healthcare Information Platform

An important precedent for EMBRACE's HIP exists in the Veterans Health Information Systems and Technology Architecture (VistA), which is a health information system deployed across all veteran care sites in the United States. VistA provides clinical, administrative, and financial functions for all of the over 1,700 hospitals and clinics of the VHA. VistA consists of 180 clinical, financial, and administrative applications integrated within a single transactional database.

This model also can be used as an example of interoperability. The Clinical Data Repository/Health Data Repository (CHDR) application of VistA is a joint effort between VA and the DoD. CHDR enables the central computers of VA and the DoD to exchange information for shared patients. Once transferred, data from DoD becomes part of the VA patient's medical record and vice versa.[4] This can also occur with records from non-VA sites that are connected to the VistA system.

In addition, the VistA Imaging project integrates all of a veteran's medical images, whether acquired inside or outside the VA, into the VistA electronic medical record, providing clinicians direct access to those images. The imaging system captures clinical images, scanned documents, motion video, and other non-text data, and makes them part of the patient's electronic medical record. Over 650 different models of medical image acquisition instruments send images to VistA, enabling the VistA to acquire over a billion images annually. Thanks to VistA Imaging, health care providers can view a veteran's images regardless of where the patient obtains care in the VHA, as well as images from the DoD.[5]

The VistA electronic health care record has been widely credited with reforming the VA health care system, improving safety and efficiency substantially. The results have spurred a national impetus to adopt electronic medical records similar to VistA nationwide.

Although the EMBRACE HIP will likely require a different underlying infrastructure, the concepts of interoperability, image availability, and centralized storage would be similar to the VistA. In addition, the HIP would allow the NMB to have access to collective data about its patients, the same way VistA is used to monitor the health of veterans.

Precedents for the National Medical Board

The Federal Reserve serves as an important precedent for the NMB, but not just for how it could integrate the many disparate aspects of the health care system or act as a relatively independent oversight body. As we will see in Chapter 11, the legislation that established the Federal Reserve System could also be used as a model for legislation required to create the NMB.

However, it is important to acknowledge that there are significant differences between the oversight of the US banking and financial system, and the oversight of the health care system under EMBRACE, which may require some modification in the ultimate structure of the NMB. For this reason, it may be useful to spend some time analyzing these differences in more detail.

CHAPTER 7

The National Medical Board and the Federal Reserve System Compared

There is no doubt that running the US health care system under EM-BRACE would be very different from overseeing the banking and financial system. Among the many reasons for this, one of the most important is the difference in the scientific method behind each. While the health care system is mostly based on the practice of medicine, the banking and finance systems are based on economics.

Though there is general agreement that health care delivery is founded on traditional scientific principles, there has long been a debate regarding the scientific basis of economics.[1] Economics is generally regarded as a social science. However, some critics of the field argue that it falls short of the definition of a science for several reasons, including a lack of testable hypotheses, lack of consensus, and inherent political overtones.[2]

It is not my intention to critique the merits of economics as a science, but rather to point out that some of its limitations have significant implications when applying it to run the nation's financial system. It is no secret that political ideology has a significant influence on the application of economic policy and that the spectrum of these ideologies is extremely broad. At least four macroeconomic theories have been proposed since the 1930s, which largely follow political beliefs. These include Keynesian economics, monetarism, the new classical economics, and supply-side economics.[3]

While there may be a similar spectrum of beliefs when it comes to health insurance coverage, there is remarkable agreement on the science of medical practice itself. Interestingly, the main limitations of this consensus are the *economic* constraints of health care delivery. Limited public funding for health insurance has presented the troubling dilemma of prioritizing, some might say rationing, medical services.

Although this dilemma of limitation to health services is brought about by economic concerns, EMBRACE offers an evidence-based solution: the tiered benefits system. The tiered benefits system is not a scientifically derived process, but rather an instrument to prioritize medical care through evidence-based mechanisms rather than purely cost-based considerations. Unlike other tools that have been developed to determine cost-benefit of medical care, the tiered benefits system was created to simplify the provision of medical services and to help the NMB prioritize coverage.

It would therefore seem reasonable to think that these distinctions between the scientific approaches taken in medical practice and economics would lead to some important differences in how the NMB might be organized and function, compared to the Federal Reserve System. One of the most important differences in this regard is that a primary undertaking of the NMB would be to evaluate the strength of the science associated with medical care and its delivery. Where there is need for additional science, the board will have the ability to either carry out the research on its own, or to sponsor outside organizations, such as universities or specialty organizations, to conduct it. Accordingly, a big focus of the NMB's board of governors would be to evaluate the need for research, commission the appropriate studies, analyze their findings, adopt their conclusions into the system, and then, most importantly, monitor the outcomes of these changes.

Some of these studies would be on therapeutic efficacy, some on the reliability of testing procedures, and even cost-effectiveness of certain work-up and treatment regimens. However, one of the most important of these, at least at the beginning, will likely be the evaluation of the existing evidence around the tier assignments and the commissioning of appropriate studies to fill in knowledge gaps. In short, the NMB will use traditional scientific method to develop and monitor the tiered benefits system.

This means that, unlike the Federal Reserve, the NMB would devote a large part of its efforts, and a significant part of its budget, to research. Accordingly, the NMB's board of governors would need to be organized in a way that gives priority to research and a mechanism to efficiently analyze and adopt the findings.

Financing

In addition to the differing scientific foundations of the Federal Reserve System and the NMB another important difference is the way each is financed. Most people never consider how the Federal Reserve is funded or think it needs funding at all. But just like any agency, the Federal Reserve needs funds to maintain its operations. Originally, the Fed was financed almost entirely by currency (e.g., printing money). However, over the past decade or two, funding from banks has become nearly twice as important as currency, and funding from the Treasury and foreign official institutions is considerable as well. From April of 2021, the Fed began relying on funding from money market mutual funds to finance its continued growth.[4]

This means that the Fed devotes a large part of its attention and resources to raising money. In fact, in the past 20 years, it has needed to create new and more complex forms of funding. Consequently, this aspect of its work has taken on a greater share of the Fed's job and, some may argue, serves as a distraction from its mission to "foster the stability, integrity, and efficiency of the nation's monetary, financial, and payment systems so as to promote optimal macroeconomic performance."[5]

In contrast, funding for the NMB, and consequently most of the health care system, will be from one annual appropriation from Congress. This difference in funding source has important implications and potential benefits. For the NMB, it means that it does not need to devise new ways to raise money. Instead, it needs to assess its budgetary needs and present them to Congress. For Congress (and the public), this annual accounting offers transparency to health care spending that is unparalleled in the current system. It will be an opportunity to see, in one balance sheet, how much is spent on benefits (insurance), research, public health, education, and the HIP. And, as we will see in Chapter 11, it also offers Congress a way to avoid the political blame that is associated with prioritizing health services.

Organizational Structure and Responsibility

Although there are major differences in the science and financing of the two systems, there are several important similarities between the Federal Reserve System and the NMB. The organizational structure of the NMB and its affiliated bodies is modeled on the structure of the Federal Reserve System. This includes a chair, the board of governors, the advisory council, and the regional chapters that correspond to the Fed's regional Reserve Banks.

The function of the twelve *regional* Reserve Banks is to enforce and monitor monetary policy, supervise financial institutions, facilitate government interactions, and provide payment services.[6] The regional Reserve Banks enforce the *monetary policies* that the board of governors sets by ensuring that all depository institutions (e.g., commercial and mutual savings banks, savings and loan associations, and credit unions) can access cash at the current discount rate. They also assist the Federal Reserve by contributing to the formulation of monetary policy. Each Reserve Bank has a staff of examiners that collects information about its region, analyzes economic data, and investigates developments in the economy. These examiners advise regional Reserve Bank presidents on policy matters who then publicize the information to their constituencies in order to survey public opinion.

The Fed's board of governors delegates most *supervisory responsibilities* over member institutions to the regional Reserve Banks, which are charged with conducting on-site and off-site examinations, inspecting state-chartered banks, and authorizing bank charters. They also ensure that depository institutions maintain the proper reserve ratio—the requirement for the proportion of deposits that must be held on reserve as cash. In addition, Reserve Banks are responsible for writing regulations for consumer credit laws and ensuring that communities have access to sufficient credit from banks.

The Reserve Banks *facilitate federal government interactions* by acting as the liaison between the Department of Treasury and depository institutions and provide *payment services* by distributing paper money to chartered depository institutions.

Although they would be dealing with health care, the structure and responsibilities of the regional chapters of the NMB would have many similarities to the Fed's regional Reserve Banks. Where the Reserve Banks collect regional economic data, the regional chapters likely would be responsible for monitoring and reporting regional health data. Where the banks supervise member institutions, the chapters would oversee regional hospitals, nursing homes, and medical practices. Where the banks facilitate federal government interactions, the chapters would work as liaison between what remains of HHS and health care providers. Where the Reserve Banks provide payment services to banks, the regional chapters would be responsible for evaluating regional concerns regarding reimbursement to providers.

It is likely that there will be other functions for the regional chapters that are unique to running a health care system, but the concept of regional oversight will certainly be as important for managing health care as it is for managing the banking system. However, the exact regional breakup of the various regional chapters will likely be different from that of the Reserve Banks. While the Federal Reserve Act outlined the existence of eight to twelve Reserve Banks, it did not specify where the banks should be located or their jurisdiction. In early 1914 the Reserve Bank Organization Committee held hearings and conducted research to help them decide how many banks there should be and where they should be located. Thirty-seven cities applied to host one of the twelve Reserve Banks. The location of each bank was determined largely through survey results from national banks, as well as the location of economic life in the early twentieth century.[7] This apportionment has remained unchanged for more than a hundred years.

In the case of the NMB's regional chapters, it is likely that their number and geographic distribution would be quite different from the Reserve Banks. What those numbers and allocation ultimately would be is difficult to predict. It would partly be dependent on the powers that Congress gives the NMB and its regional chapters and partly on the variations of public health and the health care delivery infrastructure in the various regions. For example, if Congress does not allow the NMB to directly oversee states' health departments and licensing of doctors, nurses, and health care facilities, then there may need to be as many as fifty individual regional chapters. On the other hand, if the NMB does have oversight of the entire health care community in each state, the ultimate number of regional chapters would depend on regional variations in other factors, such as prevalence of disease and existing infrastructure. It is also possible that unlike the Federal Reserve System, the number and jurisdiction of the regional chapters could change as conditions change.

What about the board of governors themselves? How would the NMB's be different from that of the Federal Reserve? The Federal Reserve's website describes the composition and structure of its board of governors as follows:

> The Fed's Board of Governors is run by seven members, or "governors," who are nominated by the President of the United States and confirmed in their positions by the U.S. Senate. The Board of Governors guides the operation of the Federal Reserve System to promote the goals and fulfill the responsibilities given to the Federal Reserve by the Federal Reserve Act.
>
> Each member of the Board of Governors is appointed for a 14-year term; the terms are staggered so that one term expires on January 31 of each even-numbered year. After serving a full 14-year term, a Board member may not be reappointed. If a Board member leaves the Board before his or her term expires, however, the person nominated and confirmed to serve the remainder of the term may later be appointed to a full 14-year term.

The Chair and Vice Chair of the Board are also appointed by the President and confirmed by the Senate but serve only four-year terms. They may be reappointed to additional four-year terms. The nominees to these posts must already be members of the Board or must be simultaneously appointed to the Board.

The Board also helps to ensure that the voices and concerns of consumers and communities are heard at the central bank by conducting consumer-focused supervision, research, and policy analysis, and, more generally, by promoting a fair and transparent consumer financial services market.[8]

Each governor chairs or is a member of the various committees of the board of governors. The following is a list of the committees (and the chairs), as of October of 2021:[9]

Committee on Board Affairs (chaired by Governor Brainard)
Committee on Consumer and Community Affairs (chaired by Governor Bowman)
Committee on Economic and Monetary Affairs (chaired by Governor and Vice Chair Clarida)
Committee on Financial Stability (chaired by Governor Brainard)
Committee on Federal Reserve Bank Affairs (chaired by Governor Brainard)
Committee on Supervision and Regulation (members: Governors Quarles, Brainard, and Bowman)
Subcommittee on Smaller Regional and Community Banking (chaired by Governor Bowman)
Committee on Payments, Clearing, and Settlement (chaired by Governor Brainard)

Although the NMB's board of governors would have a similar structure, there likely would be several key differences. The first is how the governors are chosen. While the Fed's governors are chosen by the president and approved by Congress, it would probably be better to have the chair of the NMB (who is appointed by the president and approved by Congress for a five-year term) appoint the governors. Not only would this reduce the politicization of the board but also give the chair the opportunity to pick governors who the chair feels are qualified for the job and with whom he/she can work.

Another likely difference would be that the governors would be picked to chair specific committees and therefore would require expertise pertinent to that committee's responsibilities. The committees likely would include, public health, drugs and devices, health care system research, tier system administration (which would include subcommittees on public benefits [insurance], private benefits, and guideline development), patient-centered care, medical and nursing credentialing, hospital oversight, veterans' health care administration, HIP administration, medical imaging standardization and oversight, medical laboratory administration, post-graduate medical education, and others as needed.

Another committee that should probably be included under the NMB's board of governors is the committee of the regional chapters. This relationship contrasts with the Federal Reserve's Federal Open Market Committee (FOMC), which is considered to be outside the Fed's board. The FOMC was created in the Banking Act of 1933 (commonly called Glass-Steagall), and then updated with the Banking Act of 1935, in an effort to standardize monitory policy over the twelve Reserve Banks.[10] This was mainly because the Reserve Banks were, and to some degree still are, somewhat autonomous, especially when it comes to monitory policy.

But with EMBRACE there would be no need for this type of autonomy for the regional chapters. For this reason, the equivalent of the FOMC could simply be another committee of the NMB's board of governors. It would consist of the chair (or president) of each chapter and be chaired by the board chair.

Finally, there is the advisory panel. The Federal Advisory Council (FAC), which is composed of twelve representatives of the banking industry, consults with and advises the board of governors on all matters within the Fed's jurisdiction. The council ordinarily meets four times a year, the minimum number of meetings required by the Federal Reserve Act. Each year each Reserve Bank chooses one person to represent its district on the FAC, and members customarily serve three one-year terms. The members elect their own officers.[11]

According to the Federal Reserve Act:

> The Federal Advisory Council shall have power, by itself or through its officers, (1) to confer directly with the Board of Governors of the Federal Reserve System on general business conditions; (2) to make oral or written representations concerning matters within the jurisdiction of said board; (3) to call for information and to make recommendations in regard to discount rates, rediscount business, note issues, reserve conditions in the various districts, the purchase and sale of gold or securities by reserve banks, open-market operations by said banks, and the general affairs of the reserve banking system.[12]

It is important to note that the FAC was conceived and designed specifically to address the concerns raised over the influence of "special interests" on the Federal Reserve board of governors. Although the Federal Reserve Act recognized the importance of banks and other financial institutions having a voice in determining Fed policy, it also understood the importance of insulating the Fed's board from excessive political or financial pressures. As a non-voting member of the Federal Reserve System, the FAC therefore has advisory capability, but leaves final decisions to the board of governors.

Under the EMBRACE system, the advisory panel would represent health care special interest groups, such as the pharmaceutical industry, medical device companies, private insurance firms, businesses, religious groups, and others. As they make up an important part of the US economy and are the impetus for many health care innovations, it is important that these groups are represented in the deliberations of the governors. However, as with the Federal Reserve System, it is also important that there is a distinct separation between these groups' economic and political interests and the interests of an independent health care system.

The specifics of how this panel would be organized and its exact relationship with the board would be determined by the board of governors. But it is likely that there would be a concerted effort to separate the science from the business and political aspect as much as possible.

One example is with the pharmaceutical and device companies. Although there is already a theoretical separation between the research and development side of these companies from their sales side, under EMBRACE this partition would be more codified in its dealing with the NMB. The science-based side of these corporations would be encouraged to join the NMB's committees that deal with research and therapeutics, while the sales and finance aspects would be represented on the advisory panel.

Groups that advocate for patients and consumers, health care providers, and health care facilities may also have dual representation. This would separate their education and servicing efforts from their political activities, similar to the way the tax code separates not-for-profit organizations based on their activity. Many of these groups have both a purely educational and member service divisions and separate advocacy divisions. For example, AARP is a 501(c)(4) organization that allows it to lobby Congress and state governments if that lobbying is aligned with its social mission.[13] On the other hand, the AARP Foundation is a 501(c)(3) corporation that engages in scientific research (diseases), sponsors scientific research for industry, and provides services for the aged.[14]

A similar distinction can be made with groups advocating for patients, health care providers, and health care facilities that also conduct education and research. Representatives from the departments that would deal with lobbying the NMB would sit on the advisory panel, while individuals from departments concerned with education, research, and direct services to patients and consumers would be invited to sit on the various committees of the NMB.

A New Health Care System Infrastructure

Together, the NMB's board of governors, the advisory panel, and the regional chapters would create a new health care system infrastructure that is streamlined, efficient, relatively insulated from political and financial influence, and built around science. Its underlying framework would follow that of the Federal Reserve System but with some distinctions in function necessitated by the differences between the nation's health care system and its banking and financial system. And, with the help of the HIP, the NMB is specifically designed to incorporate the tiered benefit system to optimize the functioning of the new system.

These three principal innovations of the EMBRACE proposal—tiered benefits, the HIP, and the NMB—make up the basic ingredients of the new health care system. But, as with any good recipe, one must understand how these ingredients work together to create the new system: How would all these components affect the delivery of patient care and services? How would they work together to improve outcomes and reduce costs? How would the new system create a modern infrastructure that streamlines patient care and fosters innovations? What would be the new system's impact?

CHAPTER 8

Anticipated Impact on Health, Health Care, Business, Innovation, and Government

What impact will EMBRACE have? As Yogi Berra famously said, "It's tough to make predictions, especially about the future." When it comes to EMBRACE, however, there are certainly some advances that we can expect. If fully implemented, it would have a notable impact on public health, society, clinicians, hospitals, and the health of individual Americans. The new health care system could also have beneficial effects on the nation's economy, businesses, and even government.

Impact on Public Health

The effect of EMBRACE on the nation's public health would be far reaching. This is not simply because it assures universal coverage and would help keep health care costs under control, which has been the focus of prior reform efforts. EMBRACE would also significantly emphasize prevention and treatment of the most life-threatening ailments. And, when fully implemented, EMBRACE would have the mechanisms in place not only to develop and implement clinically useful testing protocols and therapies but also to monitor their usefulness, efficiency, and effectiveness in a timely way. In addition, near real-time national data would be available on new illness outbreaks, which currently might take months or years to identify due to the lack of a national clinical data platform.

The need to quickly identify disease outbreaks became apparent during the COVID-19 pandemic. Even with the heightened vigilance in the early months of the outbreak with the knowledge that the virus might spread from China into the United States, it took weeks to identify some of the pockets of domestic cases outside of hospitals (i.e., medical offices and nursing homes). This is because these reports depended on health care professionals being able to identify a disease that they had never previously encountered and that had a range of manifestations that were not yet well defined, and then report this to the CDC. If instead, each of these individual cases were accrued in a central database, such as EMBRACE's HIP, and analyzed in real time by a computer program that monitors health patterns, we might have been able to identify these pockets much earlier and contain them.

As the brain and heart of the nation's new health care system, EMBRACE's NMB would be given a mission "To promote the health of each and every person in the United States of America." The importance of having this unifying organization and mission statement cannot be overstated or repeated enough. Currently, there is no such authoritative body nor such an infrastructure. The NMB's oversight of all aspects of the system would ensure health care delivery to the entire population. The fully integrated system under HIP would facilitate the use of practice guidelines at the point of care and allow for the collection of almost instantaneous epidemiologic data. This information would be complete (as information from the entire population would be transmitted via the HIP) and instantly available for analysis. And, when there is a need for more reliable data for guidelines and tier assignments, the NMB would have the ability to prioritize research to make health care delivery more effective and efficient.

It will be expensive to design and build the HIP, but once it is operational, costs should be low relative to the cost of getting similar information in the current environment. This might lead to substantial savings in the long run. Because the NMB will oversee the entire database of health records, the information would be more readily available for more meaningful and reliable analysis. The NMB could use this database not only to monitor epidemics, but also treatment side effects from medication and medical devices. It would also be used to modify tier assignments and even look for patterns of tier-system abuse.

In addition, because the NMB will assign conditions to specific tiers, it would be able to include diagnosis and treatment guidelines with those assignments in a way that does not interfere with clinicians' workflow and allows them to tailor work-up and therapy to the patient's needs. This mechanism of guideline integration into the HIP's Universal Billing Form would also allow for the seamless incorporation of preventive services into the workflow. And because Tier 1 covers all these preventive and lifesaving services, they will be readily available to the patient with no out-of-pocket cost.

Other preventive services and programs can also be established under EMBRACE. An example would be a program that awards Tier 2 upgrades to patients who have met several of their treatment or prevention goals. For example, those who stop smoking might be awarded Tier 2 coverage as long as they continue to refrain from smoking. Of course, significant operational details would have to be worked out, such as a mechanism for verifying tobacco abstinence. Other examples where achieving goals might lead to Tier 2 benefits could include weight loss and diabetes control.

Another possible initiative of the EMBRACE system would provide tax benefits for businesses that develop effective fitness or prevention programs for their employees. Although this might exist now in some corporations, there is no mechanism in our current system to study the effectiveness of these programs or to compare them. Under EMBRACE, comparative effectiveness studies would be much easier to conduct because all participants are automatically included in the EMBRACE database.

The NMB's direct oversight of the HIP would not only allow it to change tier assignments readily as new information becomes available but would also provide researchers and epidemiologists instant access to the data generated by the HIP on diseases and therapies. These data might help the NMB to identify epidemic outbreaks early on and obtain information on the effectiveness of drugs and devices long after they are approved and in public use. Currently, information on how drugs and devices perform in the "real world" (after receiving FDA approval) is acquired through phase IV studies, which are difficult and expensive to conduct. Alternatively, the FDA receives reports from doctors, hospitals, and patients regarding adverse outcomes from drugs or device malfunctions. These reports are not always reliable, and it may take time to identify a problem. The FDA estimates that only about 25% of serious adverse events related to medical devices are reported to the agency by hospitals. Under EMBRACE, all these data would be easily and inexpensively acquired on a constant and virtually instantaneous basis, enabling a robust system of drug and device safety surveillance. This in turn could be quickly analyzed by the NMB so that appropriate actions could be taken.

Automatic enrollment in these "post-market" studies of medical products would be beneficial no matter what regulatory response might be required. They would be faster, better, and cheaper than phase IV studies and more likely than the current FDA reporting system to identify safety issues early.

The most important public health advantage of EMBRACE over the current system, however, would be the ability of the NMB to commission studies to produce data tailored specifically for clinical use in the tiered health care system. These large population studies would be easier to organize, significantly less expensive than current studies, and have a built-in infrastructure to translate the findings into practice. This important new ability will be explored in more detail later in this chapter.

Impact on Patients/Consumers

EMBRACE would provide universal benefit coverage and access to medical care for the entire population regardless of age, gender, employment status, military service, ethnic group, income status, or ability to pay. Under EMBRACE, every US citizen is automatically enrolled, without a fee or an enrollment form. When EMBRACE begins, most people would be entered in Tier 1 (basic health coverage) during their first visit to a health care professional or facility. All that is required on subsequent visits is a form of identification such as a card or even fingerprints; all information is then available to the health care provider through their computer. Newborns will be entered at birth and carry the coverage for the rest of their lives.

Although Tier 1 provides everyone with coverage for the most important and dangerous conditions, many consumers will want to supplement this safety-net coverage with a Tier 2 plan. Purchasing a Tier 2 plan would not be mandatory, but is likely to be significantly less expensive than private health insurance under the current system. These private plans, like the Tier 1 coverage, would be portable from job to job and state to state.

No Longer Will Access to Health Care Providers and Hospitals Depend on Insurance

Under EMBRACE, patients would have access to all providers. There would be no in-network type restrictions on which doctor or hospital one can use. Currently, access to physicians, hospitals, and other services are heavily dependent on one's insurance (or lack of insurance). From VHA care that limits the hospitals and doctors veterans see, to Medicaid where patients can only see limited outpatient providers, to commercial insurance holders who are limited by provider panels that limit which doctors and even hospitals a patient can use without paying a penalty, the current system has plenty of examples of restrictions to access.

Since everyone would have identical Tier 1 coverage, there would be no restrictions to basic services. Anyone would be able to see their local doctor or go to the Mayo or Cleveland Clinic. Veterans would be able to get specialty care at veterans' hospitals *or* any other hospital or doctor office. A homeless woman would have the same access to basic services as the CEO of a Fortune 500 firm. Even the supplemental Tier 2 commercial insurance would cover all providers and services.

No Longer Will Insurance Coverage Be Based on Employment or Employer

What started out as a perk offered by employers to attract workers, has become mandated by the ACA, not because it is the most logical and efficient way to offer health insurance, but because it is what was there. In addition to the burden on businesses to provide these insurance plans (discussed later), there are many problems for the employee that have become more apparent over the past few years.

As the financial burden of supplying insurance has increased, employers have had to pass on many of the costs to their employees in many different methods. A common technique is to require that a larger part of the premiums be paid by the employee. Another is to offer more bare-bones insurance plans that are cheaper up front but cover significantly less. This, of course, means that employees will eventually need to pay more out-of-pocket down the road should they incur complex conditions or require expensive procedures not covered by their insurance.

Another concern with employer-based health insurance is that it is typically only in effect while the employee works for the employer. For many low-wage workers, the fear of losing health insurance is often so great that they would rather continue in dead-end, low-wage jobs, than look for another (or work for themselves). It also means that if the employee is fired or is laid off, they would eventually lose their insurance (there is a way through COBRA [Consolidated Omnibus Budget Reconciliation Act] for the unemployed employee to pay for an extension of the insurance for a few months, but this is temporary and often very expensive). This was brought to light during the COVID-19 pandemic, when an estimated 27 million people lost their employment-based insurance when they were laid off.[1] The cruel irony is that this is when many of these displaced workers most likely needed coverage, since a large part of the population has tested positive for the virus—about 25% as of April 2022.[2]

Under EMBRACE, basic health insurance would not be tied in any way to employment. This means that employees (and their bosses) would all have the same basic insurance, no matter if they are full-time employees, part-time, or contracted workers; minimum-wage workers would have the same basic health insurance as CEOs and members of Congress.

No Longer Will Insurance Coverage Be Based on (Old) Age or Disability

When Medicare was first introduced in 1965, the concept of a health insurance trust fund for retirees over the age of 65 made a lot of sense. Life expectancy was 70 years (67 for men and 74 for women), and medical costs were significantly lower. Now, average life expectancy is nearly 79 years and the cost of medical care in the last year of life has skyrocketed. In addition to covering people over the age of 65, Medicare came to include younger patients with disabilities and severe chronic illnesses–devastating and high-cost conditions such as dialysis for kidney failure. This has threatened to bankrupt the Medicare trust fund by 2026, a distressing prospect for the nation's elderly as well as for Americans with disabilities.

Under EMBRACE, there would be no need for a Medicare trust fund because there would be no need for Medicare. Everyone over the age of 65 would already be covered by Tier 1 benefits. Supplemental benefits through Tier 2 would be available for not much more than Medicare recipients now pay out-of-pocket for deductibles, co-pays, and Medicare supplemental insurance (Medigap).

For those who have disabilities like kidney problems requiring dialysis, most would be covered by Tier 1 benefits, and those not covered would be able to purchase it through Tier 2, possibly at a reduced price (either by the NMB controlling the premium or with premium support).

No Longer Will Insurance Coverage Be Based on (Young) Age and Poverty

Medicaid was first established in 1965 to offer medical services to the poor but was expanded in 1997 to provide insurance coverage to uninsured, low-income children of families above Medicaid income eligibility thresholds. Unlike Medicare, primarily a federal program, Medicaid is a hybrid federal and state program. The federal government pays states for a specified percentage of program expenditures, called the Federal Medical Assistance Percentage. States must ensure they can fund their share of Medicaid expenditures for the care and services available under their state plan. This means that Medicaid coverage can vary significantly from state to state. It also means that Medicaid funding becomes a burden for each state. Unlike the federal government, which can run deficits, almost all states have legal requirements to run balanced budgets. This means that there are often pressures on the state government to reduce Medicaid spending, which in turn may result in reduced benefits or the number of people covered.

Under EMBRACE, there would be no fiscal obligations for states to cover Tier 1 expenses. To what degree supplemental Tier 2 coverage for the poor and for children would be financed (if at all) would need to be decided by Congress. But everyone would be covered by Tier 1.

No Longer Will Insurance Coverage Be Based on Prior Military Service

Although it makes sense to have specialized hospitals and clinics for ex-servicepeople, coverage for these services do not have to be limited to only these services. The current VHA coverage limits the veteran to services provided by VHA hospitals and clinics. Any coverage for outside service is either limited or nonexistent. This has led to issues of health care access, especially for veterans living in rural areas.

Under EMBRACE, all veterans and active service members would have the same Tier 1 coverage as the rest of the population. In addition, the NMB would create Tier 2 supplement benefits specifically for servicepeople and veterans. Most likely this would be underwritten by the DoD (in the case of active service members) or the VA (for veterans). Veterans' access to VHA hospitals and clinics would remain unchanged, but they would also be able to access all other hospitals, clinics, physicians, and services for Tier 1 services without the current limitations.

No Longer Will Insurance Coverage Be Based on Ethnic Origin

How the United States managed to develop a completely separate health plan for Native Americans is a story in itself. There is no doubt that this population has many specific health care needs, but the separate health system created for them actually isolates them more from the rest of the country.

There are many more subtle forms of ethnic and economic disparities in the US health care system. The most important and most prevalent among these is the Medicaid program, which significantly expanded under the ACA. As of March 2020, 71.6 million individuals were enrolled in Medicaid or Children's Health Insurance Program, representing a 24.7% increase since the ACA's Medicaid expansion program was initiated,[3] and the number of uninsured through this Medicaid expansion, particularly in minorities, has significantly decreased.

However, because of its lower payments to providers, Medicaid does not offer the same access to doctors and other services as traditional commercial insurance. And since insurance coverage of people of color is more than twice as likely than in whites to be through Medicaid,[4] this is yet another form of ethnic disparity that continues to grow, even as we increase the number of people covered.

Under EMBRACE, Tier 1 benefits would cover all basic services whether provided on the reservation or elsewhere. The NMB would then create, and the Bureau of Indian Affairs would likely underwrite, Tier 2 benefits specifically for the Native American population. Because everyone will have Tier 1 services, and both Tier 1 and Tier 2 coverage requires universal acceptance by the provider (i.e., any physician, hospital, or other health care provider that is enrolled in Tier 1 is required to take Tier 2 insurance coverage), there will be no variability in access based on insurance. Other barriers, such as geography and cultural traditions may still present hurdles for achieving ethnic parity in health care, but these issues may be more appropriately addressed through improving infrastructure and social outreach.

Impact on Medical Practices

For the health care provider, EMBRACE preserves most of the current system's best features and drastically improves many of the most troublesome. It also helps providers deliver the best, scientifically validated therapy to their patients with a minimum of bureaucratic and financial burdens.

Central to this asset of the EMBRACE model is the HIP and its provider interface, the UBF. When providers log onto the HIP, they enter basic identifying information about the patient on the UBF, and the patient's prior medical chart becomes available immediately. Providers then use their own electronic medical charting program to record the current patient visit. Although the HIP is a common platform, each office, hospital, and nursing facility would provide its own form of electronic medical records (EMRs) that comply with HIP standards. Like the Apple iOS operating system, application developers will be able to develop apps and hardware that seamlessly integrate with the HIP. These apps may include EMRs, lab reports, or software to view imaging tests such as echocardiograms or MRIs. They may also include personal health record apps so that patients can carry their key medical information with them on their phone or have it on their home computers. And because they all share a common platform with required specifications, there is complete interoperability among systems.

After the charting is completed by the health care provider, a copy goes to the provider's own server (as a patient file), and another copy is sent through the HIP to a national server. Concurrently, providers submit their bills using the existent Current Procedural Terminology codes (codes that determine types of service) and the International Classification of Diseases codes (codes that classify diseases). These codes would continue to be used, although there would likely be modifications over time. Once the UBF is submitted, the HIP uses scientifically derived criteria to determine under which tier the service falls. If it is determined to be Tier 1, the provider is immediately credited (paid) for that service. If the service is determined to be Tier 2, the HIP searches to see if the patient has private insurance coverage. If the patient is covered, the HIP contacts the insurance company, and the provider is paid. If there is no insurance coverage for the service, the patient is billed for it. Facility charges (costs of using machines such as CT scanners and for the technicians that run them) would be attached to the UBF as well.

In certain cases, it might be unclear to the provider whether the service they plan to give to the patient would be Tier 1 (where the patient would not have to pay), Tier 2, or Tier 3. In such cases, the provider would simply add a query to the UBF that will result in an immediate tier assignment response. This allows the provider the opportunity to discuss the options (and prices) with the patient, especially if the service is determined to fall under Tier 2 or Tier 3.

There are no pre-certifications or denials, and providers could do most of the billing themselves. Providers could appeal decisions when a service is not covered by Tier 1, but these appeals would be considered by the NMB in aggregate only, and not for the individual patient.

Another important clinical advantage of the HIP is that all testing results, no matter where the tests are performed, would be available to all providers involved in a patient's care (as well as to the patient). This applies not only to laboratory tests of blood and other bodily fluids but also to pathology specimens and imaging studies. Reports of physician interpretation of imaging studies would be provided, along with a link to the images themselves. In some cases, imaging study access would also include the raw data originally collected by the imaging laboratory. In this way, the consulting doctor could reprocess the data if needed.

This ability to access the original testing data, rather than just someone's interpretation of the results, would not only significantly improve patient care but also reduce the number of repeat tests, thereby reducing costs and patient inconvenience. In some instances (e.g., tests involving X-rays, dyes, and nuclear agents), repeat procedure avoidance also reduces patients' exposure to harm, such as radiation and dye reactions.

Another important advantage for clinicians is that EMBRACE simplifies the issue of board certification and maintenance of certification. The American Board of Medical Specialties (ABMS), which oversees certification of physicians, as well as the non-ABMS boards (such as those that certify doctors in nuclear cardiology or echocardiography), would either be formally merged into the NMB system and reorganized, or be overseen directly by the NMB along with certification of other health care professionals including nurses and medical technicians. This change would make it possible to integrate more fully the process of maintaining certification into everyday practice. Providers could take online courses (offered through the HIP) specifically tailored to their specialties, eliminating the need to travel or take time off to attend courses.

Impact on Hospitals

American hospitals have both positive and negative attributes. The positive ones include their diversity and their patient-friendly services. The negatives, however, include a large (and growing) administrative workforce and a bipartite delivery procedure based on insurance status. EMBRACE would eliminate or greatly reduce most of the current system's disadvantages while maintaining many of its best aspects. First, there would be no difference in insurance status among patients for most hospital-based treatments, because most nonelective admissions tend to be Tier 1. Consequently, the bipartite system of insured/uninsured patients would be a thing of the past for Tier 1 conditions. This would not only improve patient care, but it also would reduce overall hospital and health care system costs. The need for doctors to treat the uninsured and underinsured would be virtually eliminated. Additionally, because the rules for care under EMBRACE are the same for each patient, the need for social workers and medical billers would be greatly reduced.

Under EMBRACE, hospitals would be allowed to create their own business plans. Each hospital would decide on the price of its Tier 2 services and make these prices available to the public—these are the prices charged to patients who do not have Tier 2 insurance. In addition, as in the current system, each hospital would be able to negotiate with insurance companies for Tier 2 contracted rates, which would not need to be made public.

Tier 1 reimbursement rates to hospitals would be determined by the NMB on an individual basis, based on the region, its disease prevalence, and the costs incurred by hospitals and other providers. These rates would be reviewed and updated periodically through a process involving both the hospital and the NMB's regional chapter. Reimbursement would include outpatient preventive programs initiated and run by the hospital, as well as medical education for trainees, such as residents and nursing students.

Hospital accreditation, which is now handled by The Joint Commission, would likely be transferred to the NMB.

Impact on Businesses

Although EMBRACE is primarily designed to improve American health care, its effect on business would be no less impactful. Under the ACA, employer-provided health insurance is mandated for businesses with over 50 employees. For many companies, health insurance is one of the biggest "benefit" expenditures, representing an average of 7.7% of take-home salary in 2012 for private industry jobs (8.5% for civilian jobs and 11.8% for state and local government jobs).[5] This expense is not only a financial burden for businesses, it can also be a distraction, as businesses regularly have to negotiate with insurance companies on the terms of these plans. Under the ACA, there has been little relief from the burden of having to provide health insurance for companies with more than 50 employees. In fact, as the minimal standards for insurance policies increase, it is likely that the cost to the employer will also increase. Either way, the ultimate effect is that employer-based insurance has become codified into the private sector for large corporations.

For companies with fewer than 50 employees, there is an incentive to stop providing employer-based insurance, sending their employees to the HIMs for coverage. Although this might be a good financial move for these small companies, it might ultimately hamper their growth because of the large increase in costs that will be incurred as they transition from 49 to 50 or more employees.

The issue of health insurance portability also poses a burden to both employers and employees. Employees must change insurance providers every time they change employers, often having to spend hours enrolling in the new employer's policy or in a new policy offered through a HIM. For the employer, each new hire must be informed about the benefits of the company's plan or plans, and then the employer must help the new employee enroll. With EMBRACE, there would be no requirement for employers to provide health insurance. Every employee already would be covered by Tier 1 for life and would never need to re-enroll. There would be a payroll tax levied on the business that is proportional to the number of employees and their salary. Businesses would incur no further obligation related to Tier 1 coverage.

However, if the employer wanted to offer perks to its employees, it could offer Tier 2 coverage. The employer could either buy these policies through the HealthMart or, if they choose, could negotiate directly with an insurance carrier for Tier 2 plans (that conform to the approved minimum requirements for Tier 2 policies).

Since every Tier 1 coverage would be identical and there would be no enrollment required, there would be no need for the employer to administer the health plan. In addition to the savings on administrative fees, there would also be no need to spend time and money on negotiating health insurance contracts. Even if the employer wants to offer Tier 2 insurance, these can be easily chosen on the HealthMart— even directly by the employee.

If the employer invests in "healthy workplace" or prevention programs for its employees, it might be eligible for a break on its health care tax. These programs not only might save some money for the employer but also a well-designed program may reduce the number of absences from work and thereby increase productivity.

Another important potential saving to businesses (especially large businesses) would be with retirees. Although not all businesses offer retirement health plans, about 30% of the large corporations still do.[6] According to data from Mercer's National Survey of Employer-Sponsored Health Benefits, the average annual health benefit cost per retiree was $11,961 for pre-Medicare retirees and $4,716 for Medicare-eligible retirees (as of 2012), among employers with 500 employees.[7] Since Tier 1 coverage is not dependent on employment or age, retirees are covered in the same way as when employed. The only cost to the employer is the tax on whatever pension the employee may receive (since this is considered salary). This expense should be significantly lower than that incurred for health insurance in the current system. Tier 2 coverage is not required after retirement, but if chosen should also be significantly less expensive than in the current system.

If such a plan had been in place several years ago, the bankruptcy of several large corporations, including General Motors, would likely have been avoided; the retiree medical costs for GM through their collective bargaining process was crippling to their overall balance sheet.

The benefits of EMBRACE for businesses go beyond just financial savings. Since all employees would be covered by an identical Tier 1 coverage as the rest of the country, there would likely be a feeling of shared experience among all employees and their managers. In addition, Tier 1 benefits reduce the pressure on employers to constantly improve the plan and could simplify collective bargaining over health insurance.

Under EMBRACE, disability insurance that covers items not under Tier 1 would be covered under Tier 2. The HealthMart would offer several disability insurance plans that could be purchased by the employer or the employee. This means that for those businesses that want to offer these bonuses, it would be relatively simple to purchase and maintain the plan, and for those employees who are employed in a business that does not offer disability insurance, it will be relatively easy and inexpensive to purchase on their own.

Impact on Governments

In a perfect world, it would be reasonable to say that government should have no part in delivering health care to its citizens. After all, what kind of medical training does the average lawmaker have and how much do they understand about issues of public health and prevention? Yet, since the delivery of health care is a commercial service, and since all commerce is subject to laws and regulations, it is difficult to find any Western society where government is not involved in health care to some degree.

In the US there are many elements to this government involvement in health care administration. The most influential government agency is HHS, which is a cabinet level department that oversees many public insurance and health agencies. This, in fact, makes health care a part of the government and thus makes it a political target. In addition, because Medicare, the VHA, and most of Medicaid are federal programs, Congress has a constitutional role to fund them. This funding role of Congress should be a simple matter, but it has become a major political issue that has often threatened arbitrary cuts for these programs.

With EMBRACE, the establishment of an independent health care board should reduce a great deal of the politicization of health care. Like the Federal Reserve, the NMB would be a mostly independent agency, and Congress would continue to control the financing with an annual budget for the entire health care system of the country.

With one annual budget for the entire system, the total amount will be very large, but it would replace the individual budgets for the many different parts of the current system, and would be, in the end, easier to manage. A single budget would lead to reductions in redundancy in the current funding system, which would likely reduce the overall cost.

Although it is likely that there would be robust discussions in Congress as each annual funding bill is advanced, there would be much less potential for earmarking and politicization of the various elements of the bill. More attention could be directed to the fiscal elements of the funding, which in turn would allow Congress to better control what it spends on health care. And since there would be only one bill concerned with health care financing, there would be more time to deal with other congressional business.

Another significant advantage of EMBRACE is that it would eliminate the threat of the impending Medicare bankruptcy. Briefly, this bankruptcy is projected to occur because of the growing number of people covered by Medicare (as the baby boomers reach the age of 65 and their life expectancy increases) and proportionally fewer people contributing to the Medicare trust fund. Under EMBRACE, coverage for the more limited range of Tier 1 services would apply to the entire population and not depend on a trust fund mechanism, while Tiers 2 and 3 will either be out-of-pocket or through commercial insurance.

On the state level there are several features of EMBRACE that should significantly reduce the financial burden. With the elimination of Medicaid, there will be no need for financing part of the cost of the program. Currently, Medicaid financing is split between the federally run CMS and each state. Some states supplement this funding robustly, while others fund only the minimum required by law, but either way, Medicaid makes up one of the largest line items in state budgets—costs EMBRACE would eliminate.

Another major cost for state governments (as it is for the federal government), is the cost of health insurance coverage for government workers. Under EMBRACE, this cost would be virtually eliminated. The only exception might be if the state decides to offer Tier 2 coverage to its employees, but this would be optional and significantly less expensive than current health care expenditures.

Also, because of the elimination of most uninsured patients and the overhead associated with billing, the financial situation of hospitals should improve, and this in turn would reduce the political and financial pressures on state governments to give assistance to hospitals. This might be particularly impactful in states and cities, such as New York, that have large publicly funded hospitals that currently treat a high number of uninsured or underinsured with all of the attendant financial pressures incurred by this type of institution.

Another advantage of EMBRACE is that it would eliminate the ACA requirement for states to set up state-based HIMs. This was a controversial component of the ACA that many states resisted, leading to the federal government offering its healthcare.gov program instead. EMBRACE should eliminate the political and financial challenges individual states face in establishing and maintaining health insurance marketplaces or deferring to the federally run HIM program.

Finally, one should not discount the financial and even political implications of having an efficient, streamlined, and non-governmental health care system that reduces redundancy and emphasizes prevention and proven therapy. Even with the recent successes in reining in health care costs (which are due to any of a number of factors including the ACA, recession, and various Medicare and Medicaid reforms), the US health care system is still by far the most expensive system, per capita, in the industrialized world, but with significantly poorer measurable outcomes such as maternal and infant death rates and overall life expectancy. Most of the countries that have lower expenses and better outcomes have a single agency overseeing its entire health care system—the key to these systems' success in reducing cost and getting better outcomes. EMBRACE's unification of the health care system is likely to accomplish similar affects in the United States.

First, there is a reduction in duplication of services such as the VHA's services that are also provided by other hospitals and clinics. This duplication, which is a prominent feature of the American system, not only increases costs but also may cause problems, such as limitation of access, that lead to strong political repercussions. The limitation of access and cost challenges related to service duplication were exemplified by the VA Choice program that was implemented in 2014, where VHA patients living more than 40 miles from a VHA facility were allowed to use non-VHA medical facilities. The law was intended to address the situation caused by the limited number of VHA hospitals and clinics that, in turn, resulted in many veterans having to travel very long distances to get care. After the plan was introduced, there were complaints that the 40-mile criterion did not adequately address the problem for many veterans who lived closer to VHA facilities but still too far to readily access care. So, Congress modified the requirement by changing the definition of distance from "as the crow flies" to "driving distance." This had the effect of doubling the number of veterans that qualified for the benefit. The change also doubled the cost to taxpayers since the VHA now had to pay for more duplicated services—those provided in the private sector and those that still had to be available at VHA facilities.

Impact on Politics

It is difficult to predict what political impact EMBRACE will have because politics are unpredictable. However, the proposal offers ideas and reforms that each side of the political spectrum have advocated, but that seem to perpetually put them at loggerheads.

For conservatives, EMBRACE has no individual or business mandate requirements, and it has a mechanism to eliminate government-run health insurance programs and health care agencies. The Tier 2 and Tier 3 benefits program also offers more "consumer responsibility," a popular conservative concept. Consumer responsibility can be defined as taking personal responsibility for the costs and consequences of what one purchases and uses. In health care, this might mean doing price comparisons for medical procedures and even deciding *not* to have a procedure or treatment.

Although increased consumer responsibility might curb health care costs and give patients greater decision-making powers, there are considerable concerns about its potential negative effects on individual and public health. One concern is that given the choice of whether to spend money on a doctor visit for a condition such as high blood pressure (that the patient does not feel), many might choose to postpone the visit or not go at all—something that would be even more likely in low-income individuals. This would lead to an increased risk of stroke, heart attacks, kidney failure, and other life-threatening conditions that could have been prevented early on.

EMBRACE provides an evidence-based mechanism to allow for "consumer responsibility" in Tier 2 and Tier 3 conditions, without potentially adversely affecting individual or public health.

For progressives, EMBRACE offers universal coverage for basic health care needs and universal access to all health care providers and health services. Although it could be argued that these advantages are similar to those promised by a single-payer system, there are some significant limitations that may be encountered if the United States were to adopt such a system. The most important downside of a single-payer system is that taxes would likely have to be increased significantly. The additional taxes would be required to fund services and treatments for about 60% of the population under the age of 65 that are now covered by private insurance. It would, of course, be quite difficult to propose tax increases of this magnitude, especially in the current political environment.

EMBRACE offers the best of both the current US system and a single-payer system with fewer of the disadvantages of either. Because the entire system would be organized under the NMB, it would have the same oversight as it would in a single-payer system. With the virtual elimination of duplicated services, EMBRACE would not only facilitate—and even increase—access to medical services compared to the current US system, but also will significantly reduce the overall costs of care. In addition, since private insurance would pay for a large portion of the overall care delivery system (about 40%–50%), the tax burden to support EMBRACE would likely be similar to the combined state and federal taxes that currently support public health insurance programs.

In addition, under EMBRACE, the public would have basic (Tier 1) health insurance coverage that does not require annual premiums, deductibles, co-pays, or even paperwork. The lifetime coverage would be fully portable from state to state and from job to job, and never require a sign-up (which is an unpopular feature of the ACA). Finally, private insurance (for Tier 2) would be affordable, understandable, and also fully portable.

EMBRACE will also have several features that would appeal to both sides of the aisle, including an easy and transparent health care budgeting process and a solution to the pending insolvency of Medicare. According to recent projections, the Medicare Hospital Insurance Trust Fund, absent congressional action, will become insolvent in 2026 and no longer be able to fully cover the cost of beneficiaries' hospital bills.[8] Both Republicans and Democrats are worried about this looming deadline, but cannot agree on a solution. EMBRACE offers a solution that should appeal to both parties.

Finally, one cannot ignore the value of eliminating (or at least reducing the prevalence of) health care as a political issue. Fundamentally, this century-long debate is focused on whether health care in the US should be directed more by the government or more by market forces and private competition. For decades, Democrats have pushed for more government, while Republicans have maintained that a free market would work more efficiently. EMBRACE offers a third choice, which removes the practice of medicine from the middle of a war of political ideologies. How this might affect other political discourse in the US is difficult to predict, but eliminating such a long-standing and provocative issue might help improve the tenor of American politics.

Economic Impact

There would also be many potential economic benefits under EMBRACE. Currently, employer-provided health insurance has been all but codified into the US health care system. Even though it does not require businesses with under 50 employees to provide health insurance for their employees, the ACA does require larger companies to offer these plans. In effect this might limit the growth of successful startups, as they reach the 50-employee threshold. In addition, the cost of acquiring and maintaining these plans often requires a significant amount of capital and personnel.

The universal portability of all elements of EMBRACE would also provide a significant economic advantage over the current system. Employees would no longer need to reapply for insurance every time they move to another state or change jobs. With Tier 1 services there is no need to enroll—every US citizen or Green Card holder is part of the program. This means that all the expense and effort of determining eligibility and need for subsidy, required under the current system, is eliminated.

Any plan offered through Tier 2 will have to be valid in every state without change in coverage. And, although the price might be different for the particular plan, the consumer can be certain that the coverage for the plan they might have bought in one state will not change if they move out of state.

When combined with the previously discussed benefits to businesses, these benefits to employees under EMBRACE will likely have a hugely positive effect on the US economy as a whole. US businesses will be more competitive internationally, as they compete with businesses in other countries that do not need to pay for health care for their employees. Since large employers would no longer need to pay for health insurance, this could lead to either increased profits or increased take-home pay to their employees. Either way, this would also be a positive to the nation's overall economy. The elimination of the uninsured would reduce public health care spending and help many hospitals' bottom lines—factors that also will help both state and national economies.

Impact on Commercial Insurance

Under EMBRACE, all private health insurance providers would be given the opportunity to appoint representatives to the private insurance section of the NMB. This section would participate with the rest of the board in establishing the menu of benefit plans offered under Tier 2, based on the current Medigap menu.

As is the case currently with the Medigap menu, there would be several different Tier 2 benefit plan options from which to choose. The options would be presented to the consumer via tables in which they would be listed side by side with a clear indication of the minimum benefit coverage required for each plan. Once consumers choose a benefit plan, they would be given another menu listing the insurance companies offering that plan, any additional benefits that the insurance company is offering, and all co-pays, deductibles, and any yearly and lifetime limits on what the insurance company will pay.

Insurance companies would not be required to participate in each benefit plan option under EMBRACE. But if an insurer chooses to offer a particular plan, their policy must adhere to the minimum benefit requirements in that category and be available in all states. (The NMB might possibly allow for some geographic variation in premiums.)

EMBRACE has several potential benefits for insurance companies. One of the most significant would be the reduced risk of covering the costs of the most expensive treatments, as these are most often covered in Tier 1. Private insurance companies would not have to pay for the treatment of heart attacks, cancers, pregnancies, high blood pressure, diabetes, and other expensive conditions. The potential liability of what is left to cover is quite small and the potential profits more secure.

Further, EMBRACE would offer insurance providers a large potential clientele with a predictable and relatively low-risk profile. Because every US citizen would be a member of EMBRACE, the market for insurance companies is made up of the entire population, without the need for an individual mandate.

Because preauthorization and other administrative processes would either be eliminated or carried out by the UBF system, another benefit for insurance companies would be a significant saving in administrative costs (estimated at between 10% and 20% of current costs). In addition, as with automobile insurance, the NMB may allow insurance companies to increase premiums based on an individual's claims experience. This will not only limit "frivolous" Tier 2 claims by the insured but may also encourage the consumer to shop around for the best price for a particular therapy or other service.

Most of the conditions assigned to Tier 2 are generally associated with limited costs and have tests and treatments that are mostly elective. This in turn means that patients have more time to assess whether they need the therapy or procedure and even to shop around for a better price or an alternative therapy, possibly with the aid of the insurer.

In addition, it is possible that the NMB would allow insurance companies to charge co-pays, impose deductibles, and limit the total payments made for various Tier 2 conditions (however, these policies would need to be clearly publicized when the consumer purchases the plan).

Because of these features of Tier 2, it is very likely that the potential profit margins for private insurers under EMBRACE would be as good as, if not better than, the current system, and significantly better than a single-payer system would allow. Like the current system (and unlike the single-payer system), health insurance companies under EMBRACE could be for-profit but could also be not-for-profit or even government agencies (e.g., the VHA).

One important question that is often asked is: How would EMBRACE prevent the creation of a competing health care system run by commercial insurance? The answer lies in the potential incentives. Unlike other single-payer systems that largely exclude the commercial insurance industry, EMBRACE offers not only a major share of the business but also significantly reduces the financial risk. With that protection under EMBRACE, it would not be very profitable for these companies to create a parallel competing system.

Impact on Health Care Innovation

One of the hallmarks of US medicine is its reputation of innovation. Over the past century the US health care system has developed many medicines, medical devices, and medical techniques that have helped millions of patients around the world. It has been postulated by some people that the driving force for these innovations is the large profit potential offered through the medical-industrial complex. It is further suggested that if the potential for profit is reduced or eliminated, it would significantly diminish health care innovation. This has often been used by pharmaceutical and device firms in their arguments against price controls and other forms of reform that would lead to decreased utilization of technologies and expensive medications.

But, when looking at the health care system, the term "health care innovation" may refer to more than just advances in expensive treatments or diagnostic technologies. A broader definition would include advancements that result in improvements in any part of the field of health care.[9] From this point of view, the EMBRACE system would promote a whole host of health care innovations.

The most impactful of these would likely be the HIP, as it would create the infrastructure needed to achieve the most important EMBRACE innovation, a unified health care system. HIP implementation would make possible the unification of health benefits (insurance), research, epidemiology, guideline development, professional education, and professional credentialing—all under the NMB.

The HIP would, in turn, open other opportunities for innovation. The very concept of a common platform where all applications can communicate with each other, is one example that would present an incredibly helpful advancement. Currently, the smooth flow of patient-related information is hindered by a lack of interoperability. In medicine, the two most important areas that would benefit from interoperability are EMRs and medical imaging.

When a patient is admitted to a hospital today, it is easy to pull up their EMR from previous visits to that hospital. If the patient has been to a doctor's office or even another hospital that uses the same EMR platform as the hospital, those records might also be available. But if the patient had records in a hospital that did not use the same EMR platform, it is often difficult to access the patient's records. Instead, reports have to be faxed or even mailed to the hospital, a process that is inefficient, insecure, slow, and often incomplete.

For years there have been efforts to achieve interoperability among medical records. But these efforts have been mostly hampered by the fact that most of the companies that offer EMRs have developed proprietary software with little intention of communicating with the proprietary systems of their competitors. These software programs have evolved in isolation over such a long period that it is now extremely difficult to retrofit them to be interoperable. One of the challenges with retrofitting is that there are no agreed-upon EMR data standards, and each company would prefer their own platform to become the standard. As a result, there have been a number of attempts to develop programs that would translate the many different software codes into a common set—a herculean and expensive task that has been only partially successful.

The innovative and, indeed, revolutionary solution under EMBRACE would be to develop a neutral platform that all EMRs would be required to use for data transmission. In addition, new EMR developers would utilize the platform as a standard on which to build their software.

The HIP platform would also be available for other health-care-related software, which in itself would lead to innovations. It is a concept that has worked well for companies like Apple who have a secure platform, called iOS, which it opens up for software development. But instead of being a for-profit platform, the HIP would be run under the NMB, which would be vendor neutral and not-for-profit. Some potential software applications might include electronic monitoring device trackers, software innovations that would blur the lines between hospital and home.

The HIP would also streamline benefit (i.e., insurance) distributions, an innovation that would cut a huge number of bureaucratic hurdles that now exist. It would accomplish this by providing the tier system (an innovation in itself that prioritizes evidence-based diagnostic tests and treatments) with the electronic infrastructure it would require to flourish. Using the UBF interface, every patient interaction would be transmitted to the NMB server (or servers), which would, in turn, make immediate determinations about tier assignment for the service and who would pay for it (see Chapter 6).

Along with the UBF, every patient encounter would also generate the transmission of a medical record to the NMB server. This would lead to two more innovations. The first is the concept of a central library for medical records. This library would allow any qualified health care professional taking care of a patient access to that patient's records (consistent with the Health Insurance Portability and Accountability Act [HIPAA] requirements). This means that if the patient goes to a new doctor or a different hospital, their medical record would be easily accessible to that clinician anywhere in the country. This also would give the patient access to all their own records to review and download, allowing the patient to update and possibly correct their information—a recent focus for patient empowerment.

The second innovation that transmission of medical records to a central library would permit, is data mining to identify inefficiencies and best practices that improve care and reduce costs. Data mining is generally described as a process of discovering patterns in large data sets through the use of machine learning, statistics, and database systems. In health care, there are many potential uses for data captured in the course of routine clinical care. According to research from McKinsey and Company, system-wide data analytics efforts could cut overall health care costs by 12%–17%, or as much as $600 billion.[10] This could be a win/win for the patient and the health system.

More importantly, the availability of robust real-world EMR data in the central library would support research that could uncover new biomedical and health care knowledge for clinical and administrative decision-making, as well as generate scientific hypotheses from large experimental data, clinical databases, and biomedical literature. It potentially can be applied to a spectrum of health care system issues from early detection of epidemics to efficacy of therapies and even to detecting fraud. An example of the use of such data for research was the RECOVERY trial in the UK that demonstrated the utility of dexamethasone in the treatment of COVID-19.[11]

In the current US system, there are three very important things that have hampered generating and using real-world data for research and for improving health care quality: complexity, infrastructure, and trust.

The complexity of the US system means the discrepancies of rules, oversight, definitions, and coverage make data analysis even more difficult than it might already be. Rather than accurately portraying the patient's clinical situation, EMR data are often entered in a way to ensure payment by meeting the insurer's requirements. Because of this complexity, attempts to collect useful data are equally complex and inefficient. Each commercial insurance company has its own computerized system, as does CMS (which runs Medicare and Medicaid) and the VHA system. The NIH, FDA, and CDC also have their own systems. There is no single oversight body that can lay claim to all these data.

Probably the most important limitation to any attempt to data-mine medical information is the issue of trust. Individual health care data must be kept confidential and their use should not be made available to commercial interests or to other government agencies (such as immigration). Limiting who has access to these data and how they are used is very difficult when it comes to commercial insurance companies who consider the information on their clients to be their property. Certainly, HIPAA regulations have been able to limit some of these concerns, but there is significant public distrust of how the data that the insurance companies' control are handled.

There is even more distrust of government. According to the Pew Research Center, public trust in the government remained near historic lows in 2019: only 17% of Americans said they could trust the government in Washington to do what is right "just about always" (3%) or "most of the time" (14%).[12]

The unification and standardization of the entire health care system under the EMBRACE model would significantly facilitate data analysis. The uniform rules, oversight, and definitions of the system would make data analysis much simpler. And the unified infrastructure of the HIP would make data acquisition much more streamlined. But perhaps the most important advantage of the EMBRACE model lies in the relative independence of the NMB. Because it is neither a commercial payer nor a government agency, the NMB would likely be more trusted with patient data.

Finally, let's return to where we started our discussion. Instead of eliminating the profit motive for innovation, as some single-payer proposals might require, EMBRACE has mechanisms to harness these incentives for innovation. In addition to the entrepreneurial opportunities that would be available making HIP-based applications, there would also be the potential to offer incentives to pharmaceutical companies and medical device manufacturers.

It is likely that Tier 2 and Tier 3 related therapies would be treated the same way as under the current system. That is, the drug/device company would negotiate with the insurance carriers a price for coverage of their products. For uninsured Tier 2 and Tier 3 patients, the drug/device company will have a published price list (or maybe negotiate prices through pharmacy management companies). For Tier 1 therapies, there would be a shift to focused development of therapeutics. Based on the need to fill gaps in treatment, the NMB would call for and fund the development of therapies specifically to fit these needs. The successful firm would get a prize for any new therapy developed in this way and a share of the revenue from its use by the NMB.

We might look at our experience during the COVID-19 pandemic for some suggestion on how this might work. On April 17, 2020, the NIH announced the Accelerating COVID-19 Therapeutic Interventions and Vaccines (ACTIV) public-private partnership to develop a coordinated research strategy for prioritizing and speeding development of the most promising treatments and vaccines. Through the ACTIV initiative, NIH pursued four fast-track focus areas most ripe for opportunity, each of which was led by a working group of senior scientists representing government, industry, non-profit, philanthropic, and academic organizations. The four fast-track areas were (1) Develop a collaborative, streamlined forum to identify preclinical treatments; (2) accelerate clinical testing of the most promising vaccines and treatments; (3) improve clinical trial capacity and effectiveness; and (4) accelerate the evaluation of vaccine candidates to enable rapid authorization or approval.[13]

The result was the rapid evaluations of some novel treatments, such as monoclonal antibody therapies. But the most impressive result was the development and testing of several vaccines. The story of how these vaccines were developed is worthy of a book in itself, but what was important was that there was a clear mission that helped all the different components of the health care system, including elements of the medical-industrial complex, focus on one goal. The NIH and other health-care-related agencies helped fund the project, with the understanding that if or when the vaccine was approved, it would be available at a set price—not one determined by the pharmaceutical firm, but one that would cover costs and a modest profit.

With EMBRACE, not all Tier 1 therapeutic development would follow the COVID-19 vaccine example. Another possible option is for the NMB to buy the rights to a particular therapy from its patent owner and then offer it at cost.

There are likely many other ways that EMBRACE would have an impact on the health care system, economy, politics, social safety nets, and even innovation. But it always comes down to the question: "How much is this thing going to cost?"

CHAPTER 9

Cost Considerations

The *cost* of health care means different things to different people.

To the *lawmaker*, it generally means the cost of supporting publicly funded insurance, such as Medicare, Medicaid, and the VA health plans. In addition, there is the cost of subsidizing some people who want to buy commercial insurance through the HIMs. It could also mean the cost of obtaining health insurance for government workers.

To *commercial insurance companies*, it means the cost of paying out claims. Also, since many health insurance companies have expanded their role in setting up prevention programs, it covers what they have invested in these programs.

To *businesses*, it means the cost of buying health insurance benefits for their employees, as well as managing those plans. In 2019 American businesses spent more than $14,000 per employee per year. In addition, employers must also pay a 1.45% payroll tax to contribute to the Medicare trust fund.

But to *consumers and patients*, there are many different meanings assigned to the *cost* of health care. It frequently refers to the cost of insurance premiums (even if some are supplemented by their employer or the government) and to out-of-pocket costs, such as co-payments and de-

ductibles. It can also cover the cost of buying medications, other therapies, or services that are not covered by the consumer's health insurance.
Finally, health care costs can include taxes and other fees, such as FICA
(Federal Insurance Contributions Act), a mandatory payroll deduction
that is taken out of workers' paychecks to support the Medicare trust fund.

With all these different ways to view health care costs, which do we
choose when analyzing the impact of reform? The answer clearly depends on one's role in the system.

For lawmakers, it is primarily about controlling public insurance
expenditures, while for commercial insurance it may be ways to protect their liability to pay out big claims. For businesses, the priority
might be for legislation that eliminates the mandate to supply health
insurance to their employees. Finally, for the consumer and patient,
there are many potential areas of impact, including reducing or eliminating out-of-pocket fees, cost of medications, and taxes.

Before discussing these special groups, let's look at the bigger picture of health care expenditures. This is what interests economists and
lawmakers the most. As set out earlier, EMBRACE proposes that Congress fund the NMB with one annual appropriation (excluding possible emergency appropriations, such as for dealing with major epidemics). This appropriation would cover not only public benefits but also
publicly funded health care research, tier system development and
administration, postgraduate medical and nursing education, provider
education and certification, pharmaceutical and device regulation, HIP
development and administration, and any other health care system cost
that might arise. Although most of these will replace existing publicly
funded programs, their cost under the NMB is difficult to predict. However, we can make some educated assumptions about how EMBRACE
might save costs and where it might increase them. These judgments
could serve as hypotheses for formal cost analyses.

Factors That Will Reduce Public Health Care Expenditures

By integrating all public health care benefits such as the VHA, Medicare, Medicaid, and IHS under the control of the NMB, there would be

no duplication of services and consequently redundant funding require-ments would be eliminated. A prime example of this is the Veterans Choice Act that was mentioned earlier that was needed to cover the more than 15 million medical procedures a year performed for veter-ans by non-VA providers. These out-of-system services have been esti-mated to cost more than $7 billion a year. Similarly, the IHS insurance program is another redundant publicly funded benefits program cost-ing $5 billion a year.[1]

By integrating all federal health care agencies such as the CDC, NIH, and the FDA under the NMB, their respective functions can be better coordinated, and funding can be better targeted. It is difficult to say the level of immediate savings this would garner, but it is very likely that it would ultimately lead to more effective and efficient compo-nents of the health care system infrastructure that would, in turn, lead to overall savings. For example, the NMB's oversight and direct fund-ing of public health would allow it to commission studies specifically directed at tier assignments. This would be a unique concept in health care research, and one that would get the most "bang for the buck." Instead of extrapolating data from industry-sponsored studies that were designed for other purposes (such as drug approval), these studies would be directed at investigating the treatment's suitability for cov-erage under Tier 1, such as whether or not it has lifesaving properties.

By removing the need for premium support for private insurance bought through the HIMs and state Medicaid expansion, there would be significant savings for both federal and state governments. These savings would come not only from not having to provide supplemental benefits but also from not having to maintain the HIM programs in the first place.

Because many of the services currently covered by Medicare and Medicaid (as well as VHA and IHS) would be moved to Tier 2, there would be a significant reduction of public funding requirements for public benefit programs. The actual amount of potential cost reduc-tion is difficult to calculate since we do not know what the NMB would ultimately include in Tier 1 (versus Tier 2) services. However, it is likely that the savings could be significant. The amount may possibly equal or exceed the amount that would have to be spent on Tier 1 coverage for consumers who are currently covered by private insurance. These privately covered patients are generally younger and in better overall health than patients receiving public benefits, and are therefore less likely to require the costliest Tier 1 services.

By reducing the entire public health care budget to one annual congressional appropriation, spending would be significantly more transparent and manageable. In addition, it would transfer the onus of allocating these funds from Congress on to the NMB where there would be significantly less political and special interest pressure.

In addition, EMBRACE would abolish state spending on Medicaid, would significantly reduce costs to federal, state, and local governments for health insurance coverage of government employees, and would appreciably lower the government cost of implementing EMRs.

Finally, EMBRACE's infrastructure would provide a much more effective mechanism to implement preventive measures than the current system, which in turn would reduce the need to spend more on treating preventable Tier 1 conditions.

Factors That Will Reduce Non-Public Health Care Expenditures

Although public spending on health care is most concerning to lawmakers and taxpayers, excessive costs that are not covered by public funding are also very important to consumers (patients), health care providers, hospitals, and insurance companies. And there are huge opportunities for savings in our current private insurance system that EMBRACE would address.

EMBRACE's HIP-linked billing system would significantly reduce administrative costs for medical offices, hospitals, nursing homes, and even private insurance companies. It has been estimated that a simplified financing/billing system, like EMBRACE, could result in cost savings exceeding $350 billion annually—nearly 15% of health care spending.[2] These savings would not only help office-based practices, nursing homes, and hospitals with their balance sheets but would also significantly reduce out-of-pocket expenses for consumers. It would even help insurance companies' bottom line.

Hospitals would also save by not having to provide uncompensated care for the uninsured and underinsured. Uncompensated care is an overall measure of hospital care provided for which no payment was received from the patient or insurer. The American Hospital Association reported that in 2018, American hospitals provided $41.3 billion in uncompensated care.[3] Since all Tier 1 services would be compensated under EMBRACE, the only potential liability for uncompensated care would be with Tier 2 services. Since most of these will be elective, there would be ample opportunity for the hospital to secure payment arrangements from the insurance provider or the patient ahead of any procedure.

By eliminating the requirement that businesses provide health insurance to their employees, EMBRACE would all but eliminate healthcare-related costs for businesses. Businesses would not only save on the cost of insurance premiums but also from the reduced administrative costs of maintaining the plans. There may also be substantial saving from pension-related health insurance costs. All these savings will not only help businesses be more competitive, but also allow them to increase employee salaries thereby mitigating the impact of the anticipated health care tax on take-home pay.

The HIP's common platform, which mandates interoperability and easy access to medical data for clinicians, would also significantly cut costs and improve quality of care. One example of how it would do this is that the system would reduce the need to repeat workups and repeat testing, which can be required because an original test result cannot be accessed. The extent of this problem has not been well studied, but most clinicians are quite familiar with the phenomenon and believe it to be quite prevalent.

Finally, the common platform would reduce costs to providers for EMRs and other important software applications needed to run an efficient and high-quality medical facility.

Factors That Will Increase Public Health Care Expenditures

The NMB would oversee a large new agency with many employees and, most likely, several consulting agencies. Although many of the proposed functions of the NMB are currently performed by HHS, it is expected that the overall budget would be larger because of the greater scope of the NMB's responsibilities.

Another likely increase in public costs would be the development and subsequent maintenance of the HIP. Currently, there is some public funding to support EMR implementation, but there is no large-scale public program to create an electronic infrastructure such as that proposed for EMBRACE. It is likely that these increases in expenditures on the HIP would be well worth the investment and might eventually reduce overall expenditures in the long run.

What Do These Cost Considerations Mean for the Various Groups?

Lawmakers will find that under EMBRACE costs are significantly more transparent and easier to control. The ability to fund the entire health care system, including health care benefits, public health, research, drug and device oversight, and system administration, in one annual appropriation to the NMB, instead of separately, would allow Congress to have a better handle of the actual public cost needed to fund the US health care system.

Commercial insurance companies will find a significant reduction in payout liability and more predictable profit margins since most of the big-ticket medical costs will likely be for Tier 1 services. There would also be a significant reduction in administrative costs related to billing (since this will mostly be done by the HIP). In addition, there would be no need for these companies to set up prevention programs for their clients, since these will also be covered by the NMB under Tier 1.

With the elimination of the business mandate (to supply health insurance for employees) US businesses will have a huge cost saving. For example, a business with 100 employees would likely save $1.4 million just on insurance premiums. Businesses would still be required to pay a small percentage payroll tax that would likely be about what they currently pay to the Medicare trust fund. This would probably be the only thing that businesses will have to pay for health care for their employees. In return, these businesses have employees with basic health insurance with no associated administration costs. It also means that businesses do not have to negotiate health coverage for their employees or their retirees. If businesses choose to supplement their employees' automatic Tier 1 converge with Tier 2 insurance, they will find that it would be far less expensive than current commercial insurance and much easier to administer. It would, in effect, return employer-supplied private health insurance to what it was originally intended—a recruiting incentive and perk, rather than a necessity.

Consumers and patients would likely see the most significant changes in cost, especially in out-of-pocket costs. For those who get insurance from their job, there would be savings of an average of more than $6,000 a year. Consumers who buy insurance from exchanges would save even more. All consumers who have commercial insurance would see no deductibles or co-payments on their basic (Tier 1) coverage and everyone who pays FICA tax would save that as well. Instead, everyone would pay a small percentage of their salary for Tier 1 coverage. Exactly how much is difficult to predict, but it would most likely be not much more than what most people pay for FICA now. There would be no other premium payments, deductibles, co-payments, or surprise billing for Tier 1 services.

For those who want Tier 2 coverage, the premium payments would be significantly less than current premium payments for private insurance (even those that are partially subsidized by the employer or by the government). It must be remembered that this Tier 2 coverage is completely voluntary and not needed to receive lifesaving, life-extending and preventive services.

CHAPTER 10

Implementing EMBRACE

Clearly, all the elements of the EMBRACE model cannot (and should not) be implemented all at once. Its success, in part, will depend on establishing its infrastructure and oversight before it goes live. It would also depend on how Congress writes the legislation. The following are some suggestions (or maybe guidelines) on the course of implementation.

The logical starting point is the creation of the NMB. As we saw in previous chapters, the NMB's structure can be built around the model of the Federal Reserve Board, with a chair, a board of governors, an advisory board and regional chapters. The chair would be appointed by the president and approved by the Senate for a specific term. It has been proposed that, for some degree of continuity, the term be five years, with the possibility of a second term. They would need to be a credentialed physician with experience in public health and health economics.

Unlike the Federal Reserve's board, the NMB's would be appointed by and serve at the pleasure of the chair. This would ensure that the board was composed of qualified individuals and be relatively insulated from political pressures. Whether to have a specific term for each governor and, if so, what that term might be, would be open to debate. However, each governor would be responsible for establishing and overseeing their specific area of the health care system and reporting to the chair.

It is difficult to be sure of all the potential governorships that might eventually be created, but there are a few that are very likely to be needed, especially when the system is first being set up. A key position would be the Governor of Tiered Benefits (although it might eventually get a sexier name). One of their first roles would be to compile several evidence-based lists. One list might be of conditions that are life-threatening and a second a list of conditions that affect quality of life. A more difficult job would be compiling an evidence-based list of services (medications, surgeries, and other therapies) that are life-extending or preventive and a separate list of services that improve quality of life. Finally, there would need to be lists of testing protocols for Tier 1 and Tier 2 services. These lists of tests might be challenging at first, since the science for testing for tier assignments would need to be established.

This brings us to another responsibility for the Governor of Tiered Benefits: to determine what data are needed to improve the tier assignments. This is a kind of wish list of potential studies that need to be undertaken to optimize the science behind the tier assignments. As we discussed previously, current clinical guidelines are not designed for tier assignments, and even if they were, most are based on less-than-ideal science (such as expert opinion). This wish list of essential information would then be submitted to the Governor of Research and Development.

Finally, the Governor of Tiered Benefits would oversee the development of the Tier 2 menu of plans and the creation of the health care marketplace or the HealthMart. How the HealthMart might be organized and operate has not been fully formulated, but it would likely be based on Medicare's Medigap program, which has a proven track record since it was first introduced in the early 1990s. The Governor of Tiered Benefits would work with representatives of commercial insurance companies to develop the HealthMart menu of Tier 2 plans. Working with a long-standing and popular program like Medigap would make it easier to create and roll out this new program.

The Governor of Research and Development would have oversight of all publicly funded research as well as commercial research related to pharmaceuticals and medical devices. This governorship would have the ability to commission research on specific subjects that are directly related to tier assignments. It would also oversee research for approval of medicines and devices (including Phase IV studies on already approved drugs and devices).

Other governorships that are likely to be included in the initial phase of implementation are those for Disease Control and Prevention, Drugs and Devices (and possibly nutrition), Medical Credentialing, Budget and Management, Regional Liaison, and Health Information. Another possible governorship would act as a liaison between the NMB and what may remain of HHS. This connection would parallel the relationship between the Federal Reserve Bank and the Department of the Treasury. The need for such representation was underlined during the COVID-19 pandemic, when there were certain measures taken by the federal government to help public health efforts. These included having the Army Corp of Engineers build temporary COVID hospitals for anticipated overflow as well as their obtaining needed medical equipment (like respirators and personal protective equipment). These actions could not be effectively done by the NMB and would need assistance from other federal entities. This assistance can come from what remains of HHS, which would be well situated in the president's cabinet, but other mechanisms might be worked out by Congress when crafting the legislation forming the NMB.

Along with the creation of the board of governors, the chair would be responsible for the creation of the advisory board. The advisory board would be made up of representatives from all the health care special interest groups. Some of the most obvious members would be the business aspect of the pharmaceutical industry, the business aspects of commercial insurance providers, business aspects of physician, nursing, hospital, and allied medical groups. The exact makeup of the advisory board would be decided by the chair and could be modified as they see the need.

Because many health issues can vary across regions, the board would oversee the creation of several regional chapters. The number of these chapters would depend on need and regional concerns. It is important to emphasize that the allocation of regions should be based on public health as well as state-specific needs.

Once the NMB is established, and before the system goes live, it would have many important tasks to accomplish. It would have to oversee the creation of the tiered benefit system and create and oversee the Tier 2 (private insurance) menu of choices. It would need to certify and oversee all hospitals, extended care facilities (such as nursing homes) and hospices, as well as credential and oversee all health care professionals. It would need to establish criteria and oversight for research funding, pharmaceutical and device development, and public health monitoring. And it would need to establish and oversee the HIP.

The HIP will be a key component of the infrastructure for the new system. There are some well-validated concepts and models that can be used to create the framework needed for the new health care system. One of the key ideas is the concept of a closed internet. This means that all the activity and data storage would be isolated from the public internet behind a firewall. To establish the HIP, the NMB would create and oversee a collection of servers that it will exclusively control. The data stored would function primarily as a library of patient charts and testing. However, these data can also be used for monitoring public health, identifying medication and device safety, and other data mining activities. Another important element of the HIP is the need for an extraordinary amount of data storage and processing speed. In the past, this was a hinderance to a project of the magnitude that EMBRACE proposes. However, it is clear that this is now not just a possibility but a reality. Between 2010 and 2019 digital data generation has increased from 2 to 41 zetabytes,[1] and data storage, processing speeds, and internet speeds have had similar growth. It is unknown exactly how much data generation and storage would be needed for the HIP, but it is likely that it would be well within the current digital technological capabilities.

This initial phase of infrastructure creation (the NMB and HIP) may take several years–anywhere from three to five (and possibly more). During this time, the existing health care system, such as it is, will continue to operate. However, once the NMB is fully established, the transfer and integration of the many components of HHS should begin.

The NIH and AHRQ would probably be the first to be moved and integrated. Much of the research would likely be directed toward establishing clinical guidelines based on the tier system concept. This would be a major change in the approach to health care research and may need a few years to become fully operational.

The FDA would also likely be transitioned early on in the process, as many of the medications and devices would need to be evaluated for the tier system. Does a drug or device reduce mortality or prevent a life-threatening condition, and hence should be included in Tier 1? If multiple therapies exist for the same condition, which is most effective and safest for the various groups? These data are not likely to be available right away and would likely require some further research than just the current requirements for FDA approval.

Once the HIP component of the system is operational (but prior to the go-live date), clinicians would begin sharing their EMRs with the NMB's server(s). How this is accomplished will need to be worked out by the NMB but would likely need to be done in parallel with the clinician's usual practice. Hopefully, EMR vendors will have retooled their software to comply with the HIP standards and allow for this EMR transmission with minimal burden to the clinician.

The final step in the transition process would be for the ending of all existing insurance plans. This would likely be left to the go-live date. On this date, all forms of insurance, whether commercial or public, would cease to exist. Everyone would be automatically covered by Tier 1 benefits that would apply at the next encounter with a health care provider. Everyone would also be eligible to purchase Tier 2 insurance from the HealthMart before the go-live date.

The concept of medical billing being done by computer was spurred by the rise of EMRs in the early 2000s, so its implementation at the go-live date may be less of a burden. With EMBRACE, EMR documentation of services such as patient visits and procedures could be easily linked to billing with little need for billers and coders.

In addition to passing legislation authorizing the establishment of the NMB, Congress will need to address a couple of other issues. The first would be to authorize the establishment of the stand-alone HIP by directing the Federal Communications Commission to establish a closed web platform. Congress would also need to update HIPAA, a federal law created to protect sensitive patient health information from being disclosed without the patient's consent or knowledge. The problem is that this was enacted long before the advent of the electronic medical record (EMR) and of cloud-based data storage. There have been some updates and additions to the law, including the Health Information Technology for Economic and Clinical Health (HITECH) Act (2009), enacted to promote the adoption of health information technology. While the HIPAA privacy rule gave patients and health plan members the right to obtain copies of their protected health information, HITECH increased those rights to include the option of being provided with copies of health and medical records in electronic form, if the covered entity maintains health and medical records in electronic form.

Now that EMRs have become the norm, health care providers—as well as systems and insurers—have access to unprecedented amounts of patient data. As a result, the practice of data mining, or analyzing data sets to identify trends and patterns, has become commonplace in health care, with the ultimate intent of improving patient care, improving efficiencies in the delivery of care, and reducing costs. Simply put, data mining has the potential to save lives and save money, but at the same time, it may run into HIPAA obstacles. In the system set up under EMBRACE, electronic patient data would only be available to the patient, the patient's provider (as an individual EMR) and to the NMB. It will be important that the NMB have full access to identifying data for all patients (in the same way commercial insurance providers and CMS have now).

Congress would also need to give the NMB certain permissions, including the ability to pay providers, bill patients, and collect from insurance companies. It would also have to assign authority to the NMB to regulate interstate commerce in health care.

CHAPTER 11

Political Considerations and Advocacy

EMBRACE is unique among health care reform proposals for several key reasons. It is the only plan that offers a mechanism to achieve truly *universal basic benefits coverage* and, unlike most other proposals that are mostly health insurance reform, EMBRACE blueprints a plan to *completely restructure* the health care system. EMBRACE also looks to create an infrastructure that is grounded on *evidence-based practice* and geared for twenty-first-century innovation. However, the most important difference is that it establishes a health care system run by *health care professionals* rather than by politicians and for-profit insurance companies and is the only proposal to address the need to separate health care from the political and special interest pressures brought about by its being entrenched in government.

Unfortunately, the fact that this proposal has so many features and advantages actually makes advocacy for it more difficult. This is true not only when it comes to the general public but also to lawmakers. It is an unfortunate fact that for the majority of the electorate, EMBRACE is too complex to be easily messaged. In the era of social media, the message is lost if it cannot be put into a soundbite or meme. This is also true for busy lawmakers.

Few congresspeople or senators have a background in public health or health care administration. Some of these lawmakers have brought themselves up to speed on the issues, but most must rely on their staff to advise them about health care legislation. This in itself is not a problem, except that these lawmakers must rely on the expertise (in insurance and health care delivery) of their team. It has been my experience that the knowledge and proficiency of congressional staffers in this area can be variable. Some have advanced degrees in public health, while others are filling in multiple roles, with health care being just one of the many areas that they are required to address.

How can we advocate for an EMBRACE-like health care system? A follow-up question might then be, once there is a call for such reform, how can we focus our ask down to a relatively easy piece of legislation? The key is to develop a strategy. This strategy should ideally be broken down into three components: a policy strategy, a political strategy and a communication strategy.

Policy Strategy

The most important program goal needed to establish an EMBRACE-based system is to craft legislation that would create the NMB. This new legislation can follow the outline of the Federal Reserve Act of 1913 in creating a board of governors[1] and giving it the powers and funding needed to create the HIP and the tiered benefits system. In addition, the legislation would have to allow the NMB the ability to bill patients and to regulate the private insurance plans created under Tier 2.

It is essential that the chair of the board of governors be a physician with experience in public health and health economics and that the term of office be at least 5 years, with a maximum of 10 years. This ensures that the term is long enough to allow the chair to put long-term strategies in place, and that the term does not coincide with that of the President of the United States.

Political Strategy

The first priority of a political strategy for EMBRACE is to tout the most politically attractive aspect of the plan: its bipartisan approach to health care reform. There is something here for everyone in the political spectrum; it is important not to ignore any one party from the decision process, as often happens with health care reform legislation. With this in mind, let's review some of the bipartisan features of EMBRACE.

First, it will check or probably reduce overall public health care expenditure. The integration of all public health care benefits such as the VHA, Medicare, Medicaid, and IHS under the control of the NMB would eliminate duplication of services. This would, in turn, eliminate redundant funding requirements.

By removing the need for premium support for private insurance bought through the HIMs and state Medicaid expansion, there will be significant savings for both federal and state governments. These savings will come not only from not having to provide supplemental benefits but also from not having to maintain the HIMs and programs in the first place.

Data mining through the HIP (see Chapter 8) holds great potential to enable health systems to systematically use data and analytics to identify inefficiencies and best practices that improve care and reduce costs. Some experts believe the opportunities to improve care and reduce costs concurrently could lower overall spending by as much as 17%. The impact of this unified health care data platform on the country's ability to manage through the next pandemic would be immeasurable.

EMBRACE would also eliminate state spending on Medicaid, significantly reduce costs to federal, state, and local governments for health insurance coverage of government employees, and appreciably lower the government cost of implementing electronic medical records.

Finally, EMBRACE's infrastructure will provide a much more effective mechanism to implement preventive health care measures than in the current system, which in turn will reduce the need to spend more on treating preventable Tier 1 conditions.

By reducing the entire public health care budget to one annual congressional appropriation, spending would be significantly more transparent and manageable. More importantly for Congress, it would reduce the highly incendiary discussions regarding Medicare and Medicaid funding and support of the Medicare trust fund. In addition, EMBRACE would transfer the onus of allocating these funds from Congress to the NMB, where political and special interest pressures would be significantly less.

The streamlining of the system under EMBRACE would be analogous to the process followed by the Base Realignment and Closure Commission (BRAC). The BRAC was an independent commission for the review and approval of military base changes. It was established in 1988 in order that the political pressures on Congress that arose when military facilities faced activity reductions or elimination could be avoided. No congressperson wants to have an army base close in their congressional district, yet, after the end of the Cold War, many did warrant closure. BRAC made the hard choices for closing military bases around the country centered on objective data and at the same time offered a mechanism to spare Congress from political blame. Accordingly, the NMB would insulate Congress when it makes difficult health care system payment decisions required to keep within the allocated budget.

Another bipartisan feature of EMBRACE is that it would definitively solve the funding shortfalls that have plagued the Medicare trust fund, because it would eliminate the need for Medicare (and Medicaid for that matter). What becomes of the fund as EMBRACE takes over will need to be decided (by Congress), but it can certainly be used to purchase Tier 2 plans for those who would otherwise be eligible for Medicare (i.e., people over the age of 65 or with a disability) or alternatively provide initial funding for the new system as a whole.

Finally, the consumer satisfaction that would come from automatic universal coverage, universal access to providers and services, and to affordable (but optional) commercial insurance for those who want Tier 2 services, will also be an important bipartisan asset.

It may be the case that under EMBRACE people who love their existing insurance plan would have to change it, but this is unlikely to be as big an issue as it was just a few years ago. The truth is that most insurance plans, even those available through an employer, have become significantly less attractive. Not only has the share of premiums paid by the employee gone up, but current plans have also imposed higher deductibles and often cover fewer services. These commercial plans also tend to restrict access to specific physician and hospital networks. EMBRACE's Tier 1 coverage will have none of these issues. Commercial Tier 2 insurance will be much more transparent and will allow consumers a choice of premium level, deductibles, and range of services that fits their need. There would be no restrictions with whom or where the patient gets treatment, and there would be no out-of-network penalties. But, most importantly, consumers do not have to purchase any Tier 2 insurance if they do not want it.

This feature is one that might appeal especially to Republicans. Under EMBRACE there would be no need for an individual mandate, a very controversial feature of the ACA (that has since been repealed through Congressional legislation) that stipulated that everyone was required to purchase health insurance or pay a fine. Optional Tier 2 coverage would also appeal to the prominent conservative/libertarian principle of individual responsibility. This concept, that the consumer should have the ability to decide how, and even if, their money is spent on health care, has been a leitmotif of many Republicans' arguments. However, implementing such a policy in the current health system infrastructure has been difficult and—frankly—dangerous.

For example, one idea that has been proposed is to give everyone a set amount of money earmarked for health care. Each individual would then use the money to purchase insurance (after shopping for the best plan) or just keep it and pay out-of-pocket for services. A concern with this approach is that many younger and low-income individuals may decide not to purchase insurance and keep the money. They would also be less likely to seek preventive services (for high blood pressure or cancer screening for example) if it meant paying out-of-pocket. This, in turn, would make them sicker and cost the health care system more money in the long run.

Because EMBRACE's Tier 1 benefits automatically cover all lifesaving, life-extending, and preventive services, it is easier (and safer) to have a component of individual responsibility included in Tier 2 and Tier 3. If the consumer chooses not to purchase insurance, he or she would not be putting themselves in any danger. Most Tier 2 services are elective and would allow the consumer time to shop around for the best service and the best price.

Republicans (and even many Democrats) would like the fact that EMBRACE eliminates what has become known as the "business mandate." This is the notion that employers are responsible for providing health insurance benefits for their employees. The ACA has all but codified this as standard, at least for larger companies with more than 50 employees. The elimination of the business mandate under EMBRACE would have huge advantages for businesses and employees, and would have a positive impact on the US economy. It would permit companies to get back to the business of business and away from the expense and distraction of being health insurance administrators.

Republicans would also likely appreciate that there would no longer be a need for public insurance programs like Medicare, Medicaid or the VHA, and there would be no need for federal oversight of HIMs.

Democrats would like the fact that EMBRACE is one of the few plans that offers truly universal benefits coverage. It also offers universal access to all providers and services, which would greatly help reduce inequities due to race, economic status, employment status, or military service. The affordability and transparency of Tier 2 supplemental insurance will also appeal to Democrats, as would the greater oversight of commercial insurance companies.

Communication Strategy

When I first had the opportunity to discuss EMBRACE with Congressman (now Senator) Chris Murphy, he told me, "It doesn't matter how great a proposal may be, it's no good for me unless my constituency understands it and wants it."

To achieve a good communication strategy, it is important to identify the key groups needed to advance the EMBRACE proposal. As Congressman Murphy suggested, the most important group is the public, or more accurately, voters.

Messaging to the Public

Messaging to the public is not an easy task with a proposal that has as many features as EMBRACE. The challenge is how to clearly present the key elements and advantages of the proposal that would be understandable to a majority of the American public. To do this we need to be able to distill the message into one or two soundbites or a slogan.

A great example of this type of messaging is "Medicare for All." Although there are several iterations of Medicare for All, the term certainly describes the two main ideas of the plan: its universality and its content. Most people may not know the details of the "Bernie Plan" that was proposed by Senator Bernie Sanders, but when he describes it as Medicare for All, they get a very good idea of what it is generally about. Medicare is a well-established American institution with more than 90% of Medicare recipients reporting being very satisfied or satisfied with the quality of their medical care and the availability of specialists.[2]

What are the messaging options with EMBRACE?

The first possibility is to tout it as a "Federal Reserve System for health care." Unfortunately, the Federal Reserve Bank is not held in great esteem. A 2013 Gallop survey found that only 33% of Americans held a favorable opinion of the Fed. The only US federal agency with a consistently lower approval rating was the Internal Revenue Service.[3] The disapproval came from both sides of the of the political divide. Before the 2016 elections, Democrats criticized the Fed's attempts to raise rates. Republicans, meanwhile, chastised the bank for its policy of prolonged low interest rates. Republican presidential candidate Donald Trump accused the Fed of keeping interest rates low to protect President Obama.[4] Once he became president, however, Mr. Trump criticized the Fed for increasing interest rates. It could be said that this disapproval from both ends of the political spectrum proves the Federal Reserve's political independence, which is a main asset as it would be for EMBRACE. But this does not help our messaging in the current hyper-partisan political climate.

Interestingly, the same 2013 Gallop poll found that the most popular of the nine federal agencies was the CDC. The public has long viewed the CDC positively: in April 2020, a Pew Research Center study found that 79% of US adults express a favorable opinion of the CDC, including large majorities of Republicans and Republican-leaning independents (84%) and Democrats and Democratic leaners (77%). Unfortunately, during the COVID-19 pandemic, the CDC's reputation suffered, as it appeared that the agency's scientific mission was being overruled by political pressures from the Trump and even the Biden administration. This resulted in unreliable (and mistrusted) recommendations about workplace safety, school openings, and COVID-19 testing (among others). Interestingly, this clear encroachment of politics into science in health care led to calls for institutional independence for the CDC and other health-related agencies, such as the FDA.[5]

How can we achieve this institutional independence of our health care agencies? All the current federal health care agencies are deeply embedded in the government, with presidential appointees requiring no health care background, and in fact often being individuals who have little or no background even in medicine or science. We can look to the lessons we learned with the creation of the Federal Reserve System, when the same types of issues of undue political influence arose with the Department of the Treasury running the nation's banking and financial system. This type of institutional independence for health care and science is exactly what EMBRACE's NMB offers.

The question comes back to how we can message the benefits of having an NMB when the Federal Reserve on which it is modeled is not well liked. The answer may lie in who would run the NMB—physicians and other health care professionals—as well as the prior independence of the well-liked CDC. Just prior to the COVID-19 pandemic, a Pew Research Center study found that 74% of Americans had a positive view of medical doctors and most feel that doctors care about their patients' best interests.[6] This would suggest that having a health care system run by physicians and other health care professionals might be quite popular.

Although there have been many surveys comparing the popularity of a health care system run by the government versus one run by a mix of private companies and government programs (i.e., the current system),[7] surveys that include the popularity of a system run by physicians have not yet been done. The reason is that until now, this type of system has not been proposed. However, it is likely that if this was offered as a third alternative to health care reform, it would be very popular.

So, the first message might be: *A health care system run by doctors and guided by science.*

But who runs the health care system is not the only thing that concerns the public. A majority of the public also have concerns about universal coverage, universal access, and affordability. As we have seen, these features are elemental parts of EMBRACE. The tier system offers automatic universal coverage for basic treatments and services. There would be no need to sign up for coverage and there would be no premium payments, no deductibles, and no copays. In other words, Tier 1 benefits would be "free." Acquiring supplemental private insurance through Tier 2 would be transparent, relatively easy, much more affordable than existing plans, and voluntary. It would follow the same process that Medicare recipients have under Medigap to find the right plan and the right price. All the plans, whether Tier 1 or Tier 2, would allow for universal access to health care providers and services. Some consumers may lament that they might not be able to keep the same insurance plan, but this is a misdirected priority (promoted by commercial insurance). What they should be concerned about is keeping their preferred provider (doctor or hospital) rather than their current insurance company. After all, the qualities that make an insurance plan good are its cost and what kind of access it affords. It would be difficult for any existing commercial plan to rival what EMBRACE would offer.

So, a possible second message might be: *Free basic universal health care.*

Unfortunately, the mention of "free health care" will only invite attacks that *nothing is free* from various groups, pointing out that the coverage is being provided by the taxpayer (or other federal) fees. It might be more prudent to emphasize that EMBRACE provides coverage and—more importantly—access to health care services for everybody, and hope that the lack of charge for Tier 1 services would be implied.

So, a more nuanced message to the public might be: *Physician led, science based, universal access.*

In some respects, this message might be too nonspecific to be effective. For one, it does not convey the message that EMBRACE draws on existing well-vetted and well-liked programs. The tier system, especially Tier 1 and Tier 2, has a lot in common with what is often referred to as "Traditional Medicare." This is to contrast it from Medicare Advantage which is also known as "Privatized Medicare." What traditional Medicare has that privatized Medicare does not, is Medigap. If Medicare offers basic benefits coverage like Tier 1 in EMBRACE, Medigap offers optional supplemental insurance like Tier 2. Using the lessons of the notion of Medicare for All, it would not be hard to extrapolate this relationship of traditional Medicare and Medigap and call the tier system in EMBRACE "Traditional Medicare for All."

In January 2021, it was reported that 87% of seniors enrolled in traditional Medicare and 89% of Medigap enrollees were satisfied with their coverage. In addition, 95% of survey respondents agreed that their Medigap coverage allowed them to see the doctors and specialists they knew without worrying too much about out-of-pocket costs.[8] Since, as we have seen, the tier system would feel very much like traditional Medicare and Medigap, one can anticipate that the concept of "Traditional Medicare for All" might be equally as popular.

Messaging to Congress

When focusing on Congress, the emphasis of the message will necessarily be different from that presented to the public. As lawmakers who represent their constituency's health and financial interests, the focus for them should be on EMBRACE's efficiency and effectiveness. The message should also focus on helping Congress understand the advantages of "ceding control" of health care administration to the NMB.

Let's start with a fundamental issue that has been at the heart of congressional debates about health care: its financing. All parties mostly agree that the goal is universal coverage for at least basic health services; they just don't agree how this should (or can) be achieved. It seems that for over a decade, lawmakers have been limited to only two options: either continued complex fixes of the current system, such as the public option and plans that tweak[9] or replace[10] the ACA, or replacement of the current system through adoption of a single-payer mechanism such as Medicare for All.[11]

Health care reform has been cited by the public as one of the most important issues of the day, and yet there is no other issue that has divided Congress and the country more. As we saw in Chapter 1, a strategy of focused health insurance reform has been the pattern followed by policy-makers over the past few decades, not because it is effective, but because it is the only available option short of a complete overhaul of the system, which is a complex challenge fraught with political hazards.

But since we have continued to arrive at this impasse, is it not time to radically change our approach, address the current organization of the health care delivery and payment systems head on, and not merely work at the margins with various insurance and taxation schemes? Is it not time to look to a third option?

The EMBRACE model is a potential bipartisan compromise to achieve the goals of universal coverage, universal access, and affordability with something for both sides of the aisle. It would allow for continued congressional fiscal oversight over the entire health care system but with a significantly simplified and transparent budget process.

Over the years since EMBRACE was first proposed, one of the recurring observations or criticisms of the proposal has been "Congress will never surrender control of health care." This pronouncement has come from physicians, health policy experts and even congresspeople. The response to this question is that EMBRACE is not proposing that Congress lose control of its constitutional role in overseeing health care system finances, but rather that it reduce the burdens of health care administration that it has taken on since the creation of Medicare and Medicaid. EMBRACE offers a mechanism to separate Congress's financing role from the ever-increasing burden of attempting to administer health policy with limited tools.

Since the NMB would be funded through an annual appropriation from Congress, Congress will effectively maintain full oversight of public spending on health care. The yearly report of the NMB to Congress would allow Congress to see where the spending goes and why. The NMB, in turn, will have the tools for measuring the efficacy and efficiency of its programs.

To this end, the plan offers Congress an effective mechanism to check and maybe even reduce public health care spending with a BRAC-like mechanism to protect Congress from the political infighting and blame surrounding health care. The NMB would be accountable to Congress for achieving the triple aim of providing better care, lower costs, and improved health.[12]

Finally, EMBRACE would also benefit state and local governments by eliminating the need to fund Medicaid, state employee health insurance benefits, or HIMs. Apart from the financial benefits, these changes will also help state governments focus on other important issues.

So, messaging to Congress might be: *Better care, lower costs, and improved health with little blame for tough but necessary decisions* (or stated more diplomatically, a minimum of political fallout).

Messaging to Businesses

For decades, the American business community has seen an increase in the burden of providing employee benefits. This is particularly true of health insurance benefits. In 2020 the cost of group health insurance averaged $14,563 annually (nearly 71% of the premium) to cover a family and $5,946 (almost 83%) of the premium for an individual. Premium costs with a group health insurance plan typically increase every year. In fact, according to the Kaiser Family Foundation, the average cost of employee health insurance premiums for both family and individual plans increased 4% from the previous year in 2021.[13]

It is not so good for the employees either. In 2020 group health insurance participation cost employees $5,689 annually (over 29% of the premium) to cover a family and $1,242 (over 17%) for an individual. Employee costs are typically taken through a payroll deduction, thereby lowering take-home pay (but making it less noticeable to the employee).

In addition to the direct premium costs of these plans, businesses often have additional costs for managing their employees' benefits programs, and many retirees have health coverage costs that continue to increase for the employer, even as the employee is no longer working.

All these financial burdens on businesses not only affect their relationship with their employees (especially during collective bargaining), they also affect their competitiveness in national and international markets.

The message: *Elimination of the requirement to provide health insurance to employees,* would be very popular among employers. Not only would it help with competitiveness but also it could allow the business to increase worker salaries.

Messaging to Hospitals

An important subset of businesses that will enjoy the same benefits from EMBRACE as other employers are US hospitals. Even if they are among the 79% who are not-for-profit, the financial health of hospitals is extremely important for maintaining the health of local communities. They also have important political influence in both state and federal governments.

Of even greater benefit to hospitals would be the reduction of the overheads related to insurance billing and the cost of providing care to the uninsured.

The message for hospitals might be: *Reduced overheads with predictable revenue.*

Conclusion

In the final analysis, it is best to leave the messaging to the public, Congress, businesses, and hospitals, to those who have a lot more experience (and imagination) than I. However, it will be important to engage all of these (and perhaps other) groups to make EMBRACE successful.

From an advocacy perspective, it is important to remember that EMBRACE is specifically designed to achieve all of the goals of universal coverage, universal access, affordability, and user-friendly interactions. It thus offers a unique blueprint to achieve all of the goals that Americans have been striving for, no matter their political affiliation.

CHAPTER 12

Questions Answered

Over the years since EMBRACE was first proposed, many questions have come from lawmakers and public health leaders that would be important to address when advocating for EMBRACE. I have addressed some of these questions in previous chapters, but I think it is important to discuss some in more detail.

EMBRACE Compared with Single Payer

A common question is: How is EMBRACE different from a single-payer plan?

The answer to this question can be somewhat nuanced because there are several types of single-payer proposals. Since it has been around for several congressional terms and many members of Congress have signed on to it at one point or another, I will use the United States National Health Care Act (HR 676)[1] as a point of comparison to EMBRACE (see Table 12.1).

HR 676 would effectively eliminate commercial insurance; EMBRACE would integrate commercial insurance in a similar way to how Medigap is integrated with Medicare. The private plans that would be of-

Table 12.1 Single Payer (HR 676) Compared with EMBRACE

HR 676	EMBRACE
Effectively eliminates commercial insurance.	Integrates commercial insurance into a unified system.
Reorganizes health care delivery by eliminating for-profit facilities and encourages not-for-profit HMO-like clinics.	Allows current diversity of health care facilities.
Overseen by HHS, part of the executive branch of the federal government.	Overseen by an independent NMB, modeled after the Federal Reserve System.
Would have oversight of only Medicare (and eventually IHS).	Would have oversight of all public, commercial, and veteran benefits under one independent entity.
Silent on who would control agencies like the FDA, CDC, and NIH.	The NMB would oversee all agencies dealing with public health, public health care research, and regulation of drugs and medical devices.
Creates a new (and mostly foreign) health care environment.	Preserves the best elements of the current system and uses tested US mechanisms and agencies.

fered in the Tier 2 menu would be transparent and significantly less expensive than existing private plans. Since these plans would still offer good profitability, there is a greater chance of support from the commercial insurance industry for EMBRACE than for HR 676.

HR 676 would dramatically reorganize health care delivery by eliminating for-profit hospitals and groups and encouraging not-for-profit HMO-like clinics. This might significantly affect patient experience; EMBRACE would allow the current diversity of health care facilities to continue but would open patient access that is currently limited by preferred provider and in-network access restrictions.

HR 676 would be overseen by HHS, a part of the executive branch of the federal government, and thus it would be very susceptible to political influence; EMBRACE would be overseen by an independent NMB modeled after the Federal Reserve System. Further, the NMB would be led by health care professionals rather than by the politicians that typically head HHS.

HR 676 would have oversight only of Medicare (and eventually IHS).

It would not include the VHA or what is left of commercial insurance. EMBRACE would have oversight of all public, private, and veteran benefits under one independent entity.

HR 676 is silent on who would control agencies such as the FDA, CDC, and NIH; under EMBRACE the NMB would oversee all agencies dealing with public health, public health care research, and the regulation of drugs and medical devices.

HR 676 creates a new (and mostly foreign) health care environment; EMBRACE preserves the best elements of the current system and uses tested American mechanisms and agencies.

What Would Be the Accountability Mechanisms to Congress?

Since the entire funding of the NMB (and therefore the entire health care system of the US) would come from a single annual congressional appropriation, Congress would have the opportunity to review the NMB's spending, planning, and budget. Not only would this make the NMB accountable to Congress but also make funding of health-care related services much simpler and more transparent.

In case of emergencies or other unforeseen needs, the NMB may come to Congress for additional funding. This would have been important during the COVID-19 pandemic, when emergency funding would have been needed for increased patient numbers, for increased testing, and for funding research.

How Would It Be Financed?

Congress will ultimately decide how to finance the NMB. However, the current Medicare funding model can be adopted easily for EMBRACE. It is likely (with some minor modifications) that the current 1.45% Medicare payroll tax for both employer and employee would cover EMBRACE Tier 1 benefits. Funding for the remaining aspects of the NMB budget (that would include funding for public health, health information and research) could probably come from a small additional tax on employers. Because employers would not be required to supply health insurance under EMBRACE, it is possible that even with this additional levy, their health-care related cost would be significantly less than under the current model.

Who Would Be Eligible?

This will depend on how the legislation creating the NMB is written. Ideally (for public health), it should be left up to the NMB to decide who is covered. It would be my hope that every person living in the US and the US territories would automatically receive a United States National Health Insurance Card and ID number (rather than using the Social Security number) when they are born or have their first medical encounter. The issue of how to deal with undocumented aliens and visitors also should be left to the NMB to decide, since this would affect public health.

Are There Any Similar Models That Can Be Used?

The short answer is no. Several systems, such as those in Israel and Germany, have some similarities, for example public/private coverage and automatic enrollment. However, the concept of an independent oversight board would be unique. Of course, in the US there is the precedence of an independent non-governmental oversight board: the Federal Reserve.

Why Not Do a Trial of EMBRACE in Some State(s)?

This is a question that has often been asked since our group first started advocating for EMBRACE. It is often pointed out that the ACA was based primarily on the success that Massachusetts had with its MassHealth plan. But a trial in an individual state (or states) has some important limitations for a comprehensive plan like EMBRACE for a number of reasons.

First, any trial that is confined to an individual state could only be done using Medicaid. This is because the other public plans are federal programs and cannot be state-run and private plans cannot be overseen by the state. Limiting the program to only Medicaid limits the size of the patient pool and of the funding for the program. This population also tends to be sicker and with fewer outside resources than the typical consumer. But perhaps the most important reason why this kind of trial may not work if confined only to Medicaid patients, is that these patients have limited access to providers. Although Medicaid does pay for most hospital services at a reasonable rate, the reimbursement rate to outpatient providers is often less than 50% of what Medicare pays and even less than what commercial insurance might pay for the same service. This all but ensures that many of these providers would not be able to participate in any state-sponsored trial.

The fact that commercial insurance plans cannot be overseen by the state also significantly limits the power of any trial for a system like EMBRACE. First, it means that consumers with private insurance would not be included in the trial. Depending on the state, this may apply to another 50% of the population that is not included in the trial (in addition to most Medicare patients).

Also, since consumers/patients on Medicaid tend to be sicker and suffer from more chronic diseases than those with commercial insurance, the per capita cost of maintaining the program would be significantly higher than would be seen if the entire population could be included.

But maybe the most important impediment to establishing a state-limited test program is that it would be challenging to create an EMBRACE-like infrastructure. It would be difficult to develop a body like the NMB that controls both public and private insurance and it would be nearly impossible to commission studies for tier assignments. In addition, the creation of the HIP and UBF that is limited for use in an individual state would also be difficult.

However, as we saw in previous chapters, there are ample precedents for most of the individual elements of EMBRACE, including "Traditional Medicare" and Medigap for the tiered benefit system, VistA for the HIP, and the Federal Reserve System for the NMB. Although these elements have not been tested together, we know that they each work well within the American ethos.

The National Medical Board Compared with the Independent Payment Advisory Board

Another question that is sometimes asked is: How is EMBRACE's NMB different from the Independent Payment Advisory Board?

In pre-ACA days, there was frustration with Medicare cost increases and a well-founded belief that Congress lacked the will to make tough decisions related to the program. This led some to conceive a process to delegate the specifics of Medicare changes to an independent board.[2] The Independent Payment Advisory Board (IPAB) was to be a government agency created as a part of the ACA, with the categorical task of achieving specified savings in Medicare without affecting coverage or quality.

It was lamented that multiple presidential administrations were unable to use the "leverage that the country's largest single buyer of health care could wield to effect reforms," and observed that "few members of Congress are well enough informed to make such decisions wisely, and some are in thrall to campaign contributors and producers and suppliers of medical services." This led to a hope for a body with the potential to "mobilize the power of the country's largest health care buyer (Centers for Medicare and Medicaid Services) to effect health system change."[3]

In 2009, Senator Jay Rockefeller (D-WV) introduced legislation that would have converted the Medicare Payment Advisory Commission, the long-standing and respected congressional advisory group on Medicare, into an executive branch commission with specific savings targets and more formal authority to implement them. The idea was to create a process modeled very roughly on BRAC (see Chapter 11).

The IPAB would have been a 15-member body that would have created a plan for Medicare cuts triggered by excessive growth in the program's per capita costs. IPAB's recommendations would have specified enough cuts to reduce program spending to growth levels set out in the law. Congress would have had the ability to accept the plan or create an alternative that saved an equal amount. Absent congressional action, the IPAB plan would become law. Its savings estimate was $15.5 billion.[4]

However, despite the passage of the ACA, IPAB was never convened. Reviewing the political events that led to this is beyond the scope of this book, but it is fair to say that it failed because there was opposition from multiple fronts. For our purposes, it is important to see how the IPAB would have been different from how the NMB would work in a health care system infrastructure created by EMBRACE. These differences can be broken down to: (1) mission, (2) scope, (3) resources, and (4) independence.

Mission

The IPAB's mission was extremely limited and focused: If per-person Medicare spending growth exceeded specified targets, a board of "experts," health care professionals, and consumer representatives would be empowered to make recommendations to Congress to curb Medicare spending.[5] If Medicare spending did not reach this threshold, the IPAB was idle—even if members of the board felt it needed to take some preventive actions.

The NMB's mission would be broad: "Promote the health of each and every person in the United States of America." This would allow for more comprehensive initiatives and for proactive measures as they occur. This means that the NMB would not be solely focused on prices and costs. It would have the leeway to invest in innovations such as preventive care that may increase up-front cost but save much more in the long run.

Scope

The IPAB would have controlled only *excessive* Medicare spending. This excess was defined by a predetermined expenditure target set by

Congress which may or may not have been appropriately set and which did not take into account true innovation. The only possible action of the IPAB was to cut funding. This means that any HHS innovation that could remedy the situation without cuts was limited. In addition, since the IPAB could not have commissioned studies, it would have been unable to really make evidence-based decisions or get meaningful follow-up information about how any imposed payment cuts worked. It also would not have had the ability to differentiate lifesaving and preventive services from other less essential services.

In addition, Congress would not have had to accept the IPAB recommendations. In other words, it would not have been a truly independent board—its final decisions would be subject to purely political considerations. If Congress did not want to follow the IPAB recommendations, it could reject them with the only limitation being that it would have been required to reject the entire IPAB package of recommendations and would not have been able to pick and choose.

The NMB's scope would include oversight of the entire benefits system, both public and private, publicly funded research, drugs and devices, and public health. It would be responsible for allocation of the entire national health care budget among the various components of the system (including funding for postgraduate medical education, health IT, and others), and would therefore be able to prioritize where the funding goes among these elements. This means that if it needed to allocate money to fund research to get better evidence-based information on tier allocation (and therefore public benefits funding), it could do so without any bureaucratic hurdles. Currently, the amount of money available for federally funded research is quite restricted and most research is actually paid for by drug and device companies.

Resources

The IPAB would have been a 15-member board composed of physicians, other health professionals, providers of health services, and individuals in related fields, experts in pharmaco-economics or prescription drug benefit programs, employers, third-party payers, and individuals skilled in health economics, outcomes and effectiveness research, and technology assessment. Of note is that "special interest" members would have been mixed in with the more "objective" members. Despite the broad representation from both health care professionals and interested parties, the IPAB would not have had the ability to study outcomes. Decisions would be based entirely on expert opinions (the lowest level of evidence), and, as previously mentioned, there would have been no possibility to commission studies or obtain follow-up data (unless undertaken by an outside agency or through HHS).

Following the model of the Federal Reserve, the NMB would be composed of a board of governors and a *separate* advisory council with representatives from the pharmaceutical industry, device companies, private insurance, businesses, and other special interest groups. This would allow these groups to advise the board but would insulate the board from direct influence on decision-making.

The NMB would use its annual appropriation from Congress to support the entire health care system under its supervision. The NMB would be responsible for the efficient operation of the care system and for achieving important patient and public health outcomes. This is very similar to the Federal Reserve's mission with respect to the economy and much more comprehensive than the IPAB's remit.

Independence

Although the IPAB has been touted as an "independent" board, it would, in fact, have been only independent of congressional oversight. As is the case with HHS, the IPAB would have been part of the executive branch and it is unclear how much independence it would have had. And if the IPAB's final recommendations could be ignored by the Congress, it really would not have been independent of the legislative branch either.

It is important to note that the reason for the IPAB's proposed independence was less concerned with reducing outside influence than with saving Congress from having to make the difficult (and potentially unpopular) decisions associated with Medicare funding cuts. The

Table 12.2 Independent Payment Advisory Board (IPAB) Compared with EMBRACE

	IPAB	EMBRACE
Mission	Limited: To control Medicare expenditures.	Broad: "Promote the health of each and every person in the United States of America."
Scope	Control only *excessive* Medicare spending.	Oversight of the entire benefits system, both public and private, publicly funded research, drugs and devices, and public health.
Resources	No mechanism to study outcomes.	All programs can be analyzed for compliance and outcomes.
Independence	Part of the executive branch. Includes representatives from pharmaceutical and insurance industries.	Independent of Congress and executive branch. Insulated from insurance, pharmaceutical and device special interest.

board's origins lay in Congress's bad experience with the Medicare SGR legislation in the early 2000s (see Chapter 4), and the good experience with the BRAC. However, the IPAB's mission was not to close military bases, but rather to cut Medicare costs, the consequences of which would have been felt far beyond the local economies of the bases. For example, what would have happened with the SGR if there had been an IPAB to take the blame for the cuts that were mandated every year? Would the cuts have been deferred as Congress did repeatedly, or would they go ahead and pass the required payment cuts to physicians (and effectively limit access to Medicare patients) knowing that they could blame the IPAB? Even if they chose not to honor the IPAB recommendations to cut payments, would Congress have finally repealed the SGR as it eventually did?

The NMB would enjoy the same independence as the Federal Reserve, with the exception of its dependence on congressional funding. This need for an annual reconciliation would give Congress funding oversight over the system and still, as with the IPAB, provide a mechanism to spare Congress from political blame. More importantly, it would create a unified, evidence-based system infrastructure that would allow for twenty-first century innovations, and would provide user-friendly health care delivery.

The NMB would also virtually eliminate Congress's need to "save" health care costs. This would no longer be their concern, but rather the job of an independent professional board of experts backed up by science and technology.

What Are the Pros and Cons of Having Doctors and Other Health Care Professionals Run the System?

If the country's legal system is run by lawyers and its financial system by economists, why not have physicians and health care professionals run its health care system?

Some have averred that American physicians "have done well for themselves" in the current system and that this should question their ability to objectively oversee the health care system. They point to the growing strength of lobbying efforts to Congress by physician groups such as the American Medical Association to protect fees and other interests as proof that they cannot be trusted to be in charge. But it is important to note that these lobbying efforts are a necessary adaption to physicians' role in the medical-industrial complex, alongside lobbying from the insurance and pharmaceutical industries. In fact, the amount of money spent on lobbying by physician groups pales in comparison with either industry.

Unlike the pharmaceutical and insurance industry, a significant amount of the lobbying effort by these physician groups is for legislation that would either directly or indirectly improve patient care. This is decidedly different from the lobbying efforts of the 1970s and 80s, where the focus was on income protections. The fact that physicians now need to hire lobbyists to ensure that they can stay in practice (and serve their patients) is a strange side effect of our current system—a side effect that can only be resolved by separating the practice of medicine from politics and special interest.

Certainly, there are some physicians and other health care professionals who have gamed the system, but they are relatively rare. In fact, in surveys health care professionals are consistently rated the highest among professions with respect to honesty and ethical standards. A Gallup poll in 2018 showed that 67% of responders rated physician honesty as high or very high (second only to nurses with 84%). By comparison, members of Congress had an 8% rating and business executives (such as those running the insurance and pharmaceutical companies) had a 17% percent rating.[6]

In addition, health care professionals have always been important liaisons between patients and the health care system. In addition to providing medical care, they often must help their patients navigate through the chaos and bureaucracy that is the current system. It is a job that has no formal training, and for which they cannot bill. Yet, it is an important part of providing good medical care to their patients.

It is this role and level of respect in the current system that makes physicians and other health care professionals the logical choice to run the new health care system.

How Might EMBRACE Succeed Where Previous Attempts at Reform Have Failed?

Clearly, this is the 64 million (or maybe trillion) dollar question! Briefly, EMBRACE offers precedents, simplicity, and bipartisanship.

Precedents

Because of a "historical institutionalism" embedded in the health care system itself, most reform efforts have been attempted through incremental change. The reason for this approach stems from the nature of a federal legislative process that is very resistant to major changes, especially those for which there is no American precedent.

One could argue that a major reason that the ACA succeeded, where all previous attempts had failed, was that it was very closely based on the Massachusetts health care reform legislation, commonly referred to as the MassHealth plan. The precedent that this program set, made lawmakers more comfortable with the seemingly large leap that the ACA represented. But EMBRACE represents an even larger leap. Not only would it bring about a sea change in the American health system but it would also require a huge leap in congressional political and legislative processes. Congress generally prefers small incremental changes, and it does not like to legislate away control of any type, but especially over such a large and complex entity as the health care system. Notably, the last time it did undertake such a massive restructuring effort, was when it passed the Federal Reserve Act of 1913. This 100-year-old legislation not only offers Congress a precedent in scale, it also offers a template for the actual EMBRACE bill. The legislation for establishing the NMB could easily follow that of the creation of the Federal Reserve, or at least use it as a foundation.

There are other parts of EMBRACE that already have precedents in the current system. The tier system can be viewed as a "Traditional Medicare for All" proposal. As with traditional Medicare there is a public component that covers the majority of conditions and services, and a Medigap-like component that offers an optional supplement of the uncovered services through commercial insurance. The differences would be that instead of being managed by HHS, both tiers would be overseen by the NMB. There would also likely be a significant difference in what is covered, with less covered under Tier 1 than in traditional Medicare and more covered under Tier 2 than in Medigap. The methods to decide what is covered would also change and would depend on evidence-based assessments rather than arbitrary assignments, but the overall idea of a tier benefits program will be very similar.

Even the creation of the HIP, the electronic infrastructure that will tie the entire new system together, has precedent. VistA, the health information system deployed across all veteran care sites in the US, provides clinical, administrative, and financial functions for all of the more than 1,700 hospitals and clinics of the VHA. In addition to offering immediate access to medical records throughout the VA system, it also stores all the data centrally, allowing for better public health monitoring and data mining. Although EMBRACE's HIP might have a different overall infrastructure, VistA certainly can offer a compelling precedent for such a system.

Simplicity

The relative simplicity of the legislation that would be needed to set up the new system is also an important asset. Unlike the ACA and MACRA, the legislation to create an EMBRACE-like system would be focused only on the creation of the NMB. Instead of having to legislate the fine details of medical practice and insurance coverage, Congress would be able to focus on the composition of the board and on giving it the tools to effectively run the new system.

Bipartisanship

It may be true that in these days of hyper-partisanship in Congress it is difficult to talk about bipartisanship, but in fact, both Democratic and Republican constituencies agree that the health care system is broken and needs to be fixed. A vast majority of Americans, when polled, agree: in a 2020 poll, 40% wanted to see major changes and another 22% wanted to redesign it completely, with only 7% thinking the system should be left the way it is. When broken down by political affiliation, there was no significant difference in the percentages that felt there should be a major change or a completely redesigned system (60%–65%). But remarkably, Republicans, Independents, and those who considered themselves "apolitical" were significantly more likely than Democrats to want a totally redesigned system.[7]

Of course, it is often observed that people respond differently when polled generally about changing the health care system than when asked about specific proposals. This is particularly true when polled about a Medicare for All plan, where there is a significant difference in response based on political affiliation.[8] It is difficult to be sure why this may be the case, but a lot may be based on the fear of something new or maybe even the suspicion that it is "Un-American."

Currently, there are no polling data for a plan like EMBRACE. However, it certainly would fit into the bipartisan support for a major change or complete redesign. In addition, it is likely that some of the specific aspects of EMBRACE would also poll well. Polling does show that physicians and other health care professionals are highly regarded for their honesty and ethical standards, while those who currently control the health care system, such as Congress and the insurance industry, rank near or at the bottom. These opinions do not appear to depend on party affiliation and have spanned multiple administrations.

As we have seen, the existing elements behind the tiered system of "Traditional Medicare" and Medigap are very popular among enrollees of Medicare; and it offers the simplicity and access that is the holy grail of health care reform.

Conclusion

There will likely be other questions and concerns raised about the various components of the EMBRACE plan, as there have been since it was first proposed. Instead of resisting this scrutiny, I and the others who have worked on this concept, have found that the process often helps refine the plan. As I have mentioned earlier, the EMBRACE plan is a product of several evolutionary steps, and this book only represents its latest iteration. It is not meant to be regarded as dogma, but rather as a possible foundation for a new way to approach reform of the health care system.

It is important to remember that the ultimate aim of health care reform is to create an American system that will "Promote the health of each and every person in the United States of America." EMBRACE is the only plan that offers a blueprint to achieve this goal.

AHRQ	Agency for Healthcare Research & Quality
AUC	appropriate use criteria
BRAC	Base Realignment and Closure Commission
CDC	Centers for Disease Control and Prevention
CG	clinical guidelines
CHDR	Clinical Data Repository/Health Data Repository
CHIP	Children's Health Insurance Program
CMS	Centers for Medicare & Medicaid Services
EMR	electronic medical record
FAC	Federal Advisory Council
FDA	Food and Drug Administration
HHS	Department of Health and Human Services
HIM	health insurance marketplace
HIP	Healthcare Information Platform
HMO	health maintenance organization
IHS	Indian Health Service
IPAB	Independent Payment Advisory Board
MACRA	Medicare Access and CHIP Reauthorization Act
NEJM	*New England Journal of Medicine*
NIH	National Institutes of Health
NMB	National Medical Board
SGR	sustainable growth rate
UBF	Universal Billing Form
VistA	Veterans Health Information Systems and Technology Architecture

Introduction

1. Daschle, Thomas. 2008. *Critical: What We Can Do About the Health-Care Crisis*. New York: Thomas Dunne Books.
2. Reid, T. R. 2010. *The Healing of America: A Global Quest for Better, Cheaper, and Fairer Health Care*. New York: Penguin Books.
3. Brill, Steven. 2015. *America's Bitter Pill: Money, Politics, Backroom Deals, and the Fight to Fix Our Broken Healthcare System*. New York: Random House.
4. Rosenthal, Elisabeth. 2018. *An American Sickness: How Healthcare Became Big Business and How You Can Take It Back*. New York: Penguin Books.

Chapter 1 The American Health Care System Disorder

1. OECD. n.d. "Health Status: Maternal and Infant Mortality." https://stats.oecd.org /index.aspx?queryid=30116 (accessed December 20, 2021).
2. Mended Hearts. 2018. "Eliminating Barriers to Cardiac Rehabilitation." https:// mendedhearts.org/wp-content/uploads/2018/01/CR-Issue-Brief-Final.pdf (accessed December 20, 2021).
3. The National Council on Aging. 2021. "How to Partner with Hospitals for Community-Based Services." Ncoa.org. June 10. https://www.ncoa.org/article /how-to-partner-with-hospitals-for-community-based-services.
4. Brezinski, Elizabeth A., Jaskaran S. Dhillon, and April W. Armstrong. 2015. "Economic Burden of Psoriasis in the United States." *JAMA Dermatology* 151 (6): 651. https://doi.org/10.1001/jamadermatol.2014.3593.
5. CDC. 2020. "What Is Diabetes?" June 11. https://www.cdc.gov/diabetes/basics /diabetes.html.
6. Lindberg, Sara. 2018. "The Cost of Type 2 Diabetes: Medication, Supplies, and More." Healthline. October 25. https://www.healthline.com/health/cost-of -diabetes#1.
7. Cleary, Ekaterina G., Jennifer M. Beierlein, Navleen Surjit Khanuja, Laura M. McNamee, and Fred D. Ledley. 2018. "Contribution of NIH Funding to New Drug Approvals 2010–2016." *Proceedings of the National Academy of Sciences of the United States of America* 115 (10): 2329–34. doi:10.1073/pnas.1715368115
8. FDA. 2018. "What Are the Different Types of Clinical Research?" January 4. https:// www.fda.gov/patients/clinical-trials-what-patients-need-know/what-are-different -types-clinical-research.
9. Liptak, Kevin. 2017. "Trump: 'Nobody Knew Health Care Could be So Compli-

cated.'" CNN. February 28. https://edition.cnn.com/2017/02/27/politics/trump
-health-care-complicated/index.html.

10. Halpin, Helen A., and Peter Harbage. 2010. "The Origins and Demise of the Public
    Option." *Health Affairs* 29 (6): 1117–24. https://doi.org/10.1377/hlthaff.2010.0363.

11. The White House. 2020. "Remarks by President Trump, Vice President Pence, and
    Mwembers of the Coronavirus Task Force in Press Conference." 27 February.
    https://www.whitehouse.gov/briefings-statements/remarks-president-trump-vice
    -president-pence-members-coronavirus-task-force-press-conference/ (archived).

12. United States Congress Joint Economic Committee Republicans. 2010. "Health
    Care Chart." August 2. https://www.jec.senate.gov/public/index.cfm/republicans
    /2010/8/america-s-new-health-care-system-revealed.

Chapter 2   *The Ideal American Health Care System*

1. Tolbert, Jennifer, Kendal Orgera, and Anthony Damico. 2020. "Key Facts about
   the Uninsured Population." The Henry J. Kaiser Family Foundation. November 6.
   https://www.kff.org/uninsured/issue-brief/key-facts-about-the-uninsured
   -population.

2. Associated Press. 1966. "King Berates Medical Care Given Negroes." *Oshkosh Daily
   Northwestern* (Wisconsin). March 26. https://www.newspapers.com/clip/12049661
   /oshkosh-daily-northwestern-32666/.

3. Himber, Vaughn. 2019. "How Many Americans Get Health Insurance from Their
   Employer?" eHealth. May 29. https://www.ehealthinsurance.com/resources/small
   -business/how-many-americans-get-health-insurance-from-their-employer.

4. Nova, Annie. 2020. "Millions of Americans Have Lost Health Insurance in This
   Pandemic-Driven Recession: Here Are Their Options." CNBC. August 28. https://
   www.cnbc.com/2020/08/28/millions-of-americans-lost-health-insurance-amid
   -pandemic-here-are-options.html.

5. Westneat, Danny. 2020. "Coronavirus Survival Comes with a $1.1 Million, 181-Page
   Price Tag." *The Seattle Times*, June 12. https://www.seattletimes.com/seattle-news
   /inspiring-story-of-seattle-mans-coronavirus-survival-comes-with-a-1-1-million
   -dollar-hospital-bill/.

6. American Board of Medical Specialties. n.d. "American Board of Internal Medicine:
   Subspecialties." abms.org. https://www.abms.org/board/american-board-of-internal
   -medicine/#abim-im (accessed May 9, 2022).

7. Translational Cancer Research Network. 2018. "Translational Research: Defining
   the 'T's.'" January 16. http://www.tcrn.unsw.edu.au/
   translational-research-definitions.

8. Stolberg, Sheryl Gay. 2020. "Trump Administration Strips C.D.C. of Control of
   Coronavirus Data." *New York Times.* July 14. https://www.nytimes.com/2020/07/14
   /us/politics/trump-cdc-coronavirus.html?referringSource=articleShare.

9. Cathey, Libby. 2020. "Trump Versus the Doctors: When the President and His
   Experts Contradict Each Other." ABC News. April 25. https://abcnews.go.com
   /Politics/trump-versus-doctors-president-experts-contradict/story?id=70330642.

Chapter 3 Health Care and the Economy

1. Relman, Arnold S. 1980. "The New Medical-Industrial Complex." *New England Journal of Medicine* 303 (17): 963–70. https://doi.org/10.1056/nejm19801023 3031703.

2. Centers for Medicare & Medicaid Services. 2020. "Historical." December 16. https://www.cms.gov/Research-Statistics-Data-and-Systems/Statistics-Trends -and-Reports/NationalHealthExpendData/NationalHealthAccountsHistorical.

3. Himmelstein, David U., et al., 2014. "A Comparison of Hospital Administrative Costs in Eight Nations: U.S. Costs Exceed All Others by Far." *Health Affairs* 33 (9): 1586–94. https://doi.org/10.26099/87pf-1r65.

4. Sood, Neeraj, Arkadipta Ghosh, and José J. Escarce. 2009. "Employer-Sponsored Insurance, Health Care Cost Growth, and the Economic Performance of U.S. Industries." *Health Services Research* 44 (5p1): 1449–64. https://doi.org/10.1111/j.1475 -6773.2009.00985.x.

5. Stolberg, Sheryl Gay. 2020. "A Record 5.4 Million Americans Have Lost Health Insurance, Study Finds." *New York Times.* July 13. https://www.nytimes.com/2020 /07/13/world/coronavirus-updates.html?action=click&module=Top%20Stories &pgtype=Homepage.

6. Kalorama Information. 2017. "Consumers Reach into Their Pockets as U.S. Out-of-Pocket Healthcare Spending Reaches $486 Billion: Report." www.prnewswire .com. April 26. https://www.prnewswire.com/news-releases/consumers-reach-into -their-pockets-as-us-out-of-pocket-healthcare-spending-reaches-486-billion-report -300444729.html.

7. Makary, Marty. 2019. "We Spend about Half of Our Federal Tax Dollars on Health Care: That's Ridiculous." *USA Today.* September 16. https://www.usatoday.com /story/opinion/2019/09/16/spend-about-half-federal-tax-dollars-health-care -ridiculous-column/2301040001/.

8. National Conference of State Legislatures. 2018. "Insurance Carriers and Access to Healthcare Providers: Network Adequacy." www.ncsl.org. February 1. https://www .ncsl.org/research/health/insurance-carriers-and-access-to-healthcare-providers -network-adequacy.aspx.

9. Tikkanen, Roosa, and Melinda Abrams. 2020. "U.S. Health Care from a Global Perspective, 2019: Higher Spending, Worse Outcomes?" The Commonwealth Fund. January 30. https://doi.org/10.26099/7avy-fc29.

Chapter 4 Lessons from the Creation of the Federal Reserve System

1. Lowenstein, Roger. 2016. *America's Bank: The Epic Struggle to Create the Federal Reserve.* New York: Penguin.

2. Tolbert, Jennifer, Kendal Orgera, and Anthony Damico. 2020. "Key Facts about the Uninsured Population." The Henry J. Kaiser Family Foundation. November 6. https://www.kff.org/uninsured/issue-brief/key-facts-about-the-uninsured -population/.

Chapter 5 How a National Medical Board Can Help the Current Health Care System's Problems

1. Board of Governors of the Federal Reserve System. 2019. "The Fed: Why Is it Important to Separate Federal Reserve Monetary Policy Decisions from Political Influence?" www.federalreserve.gov. December 31. 2014. https://www.federal reserve.gov/faqs/why-is-it-important-to-separate-federal-reserve-monetary-policy -decisions-from-political-influence.htm.
2. American Rhetoric. 2022. "Ronald Reagan: Radio Address on Socialized Medi-cine." www.americanrhetoric.com. 6 January. https://www.americanrhetoric.com /speeches/ronaldreagansocializedmedicine.htm.
3. Allen, Marshall. 2018. "Health Insurers Are Vacuuming up Details about You — and It Could Raise Your Rates." ProPublica. July 17. https://www.propublica.org/article /health-insurers-are-vacuuming-up-details-about-you-and-it-could-raise-your -rates.

Chapter 6 EMBRACE

1. Centers for Medicare & Medicaid Services. 2021. "NHE Fact Sheet." www.cms.gov. 15 December. http://www.cms.gov/Research-Statistics-Data-and-Systems/Statistics -Trends-and-Reports/NationalHealthExpendData/NHE-Fact-Sheet.html.
2. Lancaster, Gilead I, Ryan O'Connell, David L. Katz, JoAnn E. Manson, William R. Hutchison, Charles Landau, and Kimberly A. Yonkers. 2009. "The Expanding Medical and Behavioral Resources with Access to Care for Everyone Health Plan." *Annals of Internal Medicine* 150 (7): 490. https://doi.org/10.7326/0003-4819-150-7 -200904070-00113.
3. Jiwani, Aliya, David Himmelstein, Steffie Woolhandler, and James G Kahn. 2014. "Billing and Insurance-Related Administrative Costs in United States' Health Care: Synthesis of Micro-Costing Evidence." *BMC Health Services Research* 14 (1). https:// doi.org/10.1186/s12913-014-0556-7.
4. United States Department of Veterans Affairs. 2009. "VA/DoD Health Information Sharing." www.va.gov. March 3. https://web.archive.org/web/20091024045131/http: /www1.va.gov/vadodhealthitsharing/page.cfm?pg=9.
5. United States Department of Veterans Affairs. 2020. "VistA Imaging Acquires Its 10 Billionth Medical Image." DigitalVA. January 2020. https://www.oit.va.gov/news /article/?read=vista-imaging-acquires-its-10-billionth-medical-image.

Chapter 7 The National Medical Board and the Federal Reserve System Compared

1. The Library of Economics and Liberty. n.d. "Is Economics a Science?" Econlib.org. https://www.econlib.org/library/Topics/College/iseconomicsascience.html (accessed April 28, 2022).
2. Peters, Katelyn. 2021. "Is Economics a Science?" Investopedia. August 14. https:// www.investopedia.com/ask/answers/030315/economics-science.asp.
3. Sahu, Anandi. n.d. "Economic Theories." Referenceforbusiness.com. https://www

.referenceforbusiness.com/encyclopedia/Eco-Ent/Economic-Theories.html (accessed April 28, 2022).

4. Nelson, Bill. 2021. "A Very Different Federal Reserve Funding Model." Bank Policy Institute. June 16. https://bpi.com/a-very-different-federal-reserve-funding-model /#_ftn1.

5. Board of Governors of the Federal Reserve System. 1997. "Government Performance and Results Act Planning Document 1997–2002." Washington, DC: Board of Governors of the Federal Reserve System. https://www.federalreserve.gov /boarddocs/rptcongress/98frgpra.pdf.

6. Du, Jack. 2021. "What Do the Federal Reserve Banks Do?" Investopedia. October 21. https://www.investopedia.com/articles/investing/061515/what-do-federal-reserve -banks-do.asp#citation-4.

7. Needler, Ella, and Genevieve Podleski. 2021. "The Fed's Structure." Federal Reserve History. May. https://www.federalreservehistory.org/essays/fed-structure.

8. Board of Governors of the Federal Reserve System. 2022. "Federal Reserve Board." www.federalreserve.gov. April 4. https://www.federalreserve.gov/aboutthefed /structure-federal-reserve-board.htm.

9. Board of Governors of the Federal Reserve System. "Federal Reserve Board: Board Members." www.federalreserve.gov. 2019. https://www.federalreserve.gov/about thefed/bios/board/default.htm.

10. Richardson, Gary, Alejandro Komai, and Michael Gou. 2013. "Banking Act of 1935." Federal Reserve History. November 22. https://www.federalreservehistory.org /essays/banking-act-of-1935.

11. Board of Governors of the Federal Reserve System. 2021. "Federal Advisory Council." www.federalreserve.gov. 2021. https://www.federalreserve.gov/aboutthefed/fac .htm.

12. Board of Governors of the Federal Reserve System. 2017. "Section 12: Federal Advisory Council." www.federalreserve.gov. March 13. https://www.federalreserve .gov/aboutthefed/section12.htm.

13. American Association of Retired Persons. 2011. "About AARP: IRS Definition." AARP. March 3. https://www.aarp.org/about-aarp/info-03-2011/irs_definition.html.

14. Charity Navigator. n.d. "AARP Foundation." Charity Navigator. https://www.charity navigator.org/index.cfm?bay=search.irs&ein=520794300 (accessed April 28, 2022).

Chapter 8 Anticipated Impact on Health, Health Care, Business, Innovation, and Government

1. Pifer, Rebecca. 2020. "27M Americans May Have Lost Job-Based Health Insurance Due to COVID-19 Downturn." Healthcare Dive. May 13. https://www.healthcaredive .com/news/27m-americans-may-have-lost-job-based-health-insurance-due-to -covid-19-down/577852/.

2. Johns Hopkins University and Medicine. 2022. "Coronavirus Resource Center: United States." coronavirus.jhu.edu. May 10. https://coronavirus.jhu.edu/region /united-states

3. Medicaid and CHIP Payment and Access Commission. n.d. "Medicaid Enrollment

Changes Following the ACA." Macpac.gov. https://www.macpac.gov/subtopic /medicaid-enrollment-changes-following-the-aca/ (accessed April 29, 2022).

4. Artiga, Samantha, Kendal Orgera, and Anthony Damico. 2020. "Changes in Health Coverage by Race and Ethnicity Since the ACA, 2010–2018." Henry J. Kaiser Family Foundation. March 5. https://www.kff.org/racial-equity-and-health-policy/issue -brief/changes-in-health-coverage-by-race-and-ethnicity-since-the-aca-2010-2018/ (accessed June 14, 2021).

5. Bureau of Labor Statistics. 2016. "Employer Costs for Employee Compensation: June 2016." News Release. September 8. Washington, DC: Department of Labor. https://www.bls.gov/news.release/archives/ecec_09082016.pdf

6. Henry J. Kaiser Family Foundation. 2020. "2020 Employer Health Benefits Survey: Section 11; Retiree Health Benefits." October 8. https://www.kff.org/report-section /ehbs-2020-section-11-retiree-health-benefits/.

7. Mercer. 2013. "Mercer's National Survey of Employer-Sponsored Health Plans." February 19. http://benefitcommunications.com/upload/downloads/Mercer_Survey _2013.pdf (accessed April 29, 2022)

8. Commonwealth Fund. 2021. "Putting Medicare Solvency Projections into Per- spective." The Commonwealth Fund. September 1. https://www.commonwealth fund.org/blog/2021/putting-medicare-solvency-projections-perspective.

9. Kimble, Leighann, and M. Rashad Massoud. 2017. "What Do We Mean by Innova- tion in Healthcare?" *European Medical Journal* 1(1): 89–91. https://www.emjreviews .com/innovations/article/what-do-we-mean-by-innovation-in-healthcare/.

10. USF Health. 2017. "Data Mining in Healthcare: Purpose, Benefits, and Applications." USF Health Online. February 15. https://www.usfhealthonline.com/resources /healthcare-analytics/data-mining-in-healthcare/.

11. The RECOVERY Collaborative Group. 2020. "Dexamethasone in Hospitalized Patients with Covid-19: Preliminary Report." *New England Journal of Medicine* 384 (8). https://doi.org/10.1056/nejmoa2021436.

12. Pew Research Center. 2019. "Public Trust in Government: 1958–2019." Pew Re- search Center. April 11. https://www.pewresearch.org/politics/2019/04/11/public -trust-in-government-1958-2019/.

13. NIH. n.d. "Accelerating COVID-19 Therapeutic Interventions and Vaccines (ACTIV)." National Institutes of Health. n.d. https://www.nih.gov/research-training /medical-research-initiatives/activ.

Chapter 9 Cost Considerations

1. IHS. 2020. "IHS Profile." August. Rockville, MD: Indian Health Service. https:// www.ihs.gov/newsroom/factsheets/ihsprofile/.

2. Jiwani, Aliya, David Himmelstein, Steffie Woolhandler, and James G Kahn. 2014. "Billing and Insurance-Related Administrative Costs in United States' Health Care: Synthesis of Micro-Costing Evidence." *BMC Health Services Research* 14 (1). https:// doi.org/10.1186/s12913-014-0556-7.

3. American Hospital Association. 2020. "Fact Sheet: Uncompensated Hospital Care

Cost." Chicago: American Hospital Association. https://www.aha.org/fact-sheets/2020-01-06-fact-sheet-uncompensated-hospital-care-cost.

Chapter 10 Implementing EMBRACE

1. Holst, Arne. 2021. "Data Created Worldwide 2010–2025." Statista. June 7. https://www.statista.com/statistics/871513/worldwide-data-created/.

Chapter 11 Political Considerations and Advocacy

1. Board of Governors of the Federal Reserve System. 2017. "Section 10: Board of Governors of the Federal Reserve System." www.federalreserve.gov. March 13. https://www.federalreserve.gov/aboutthefed/section10.htm.
2. Ochieng, Nancy, Jeannie Fuglesten Biniek, Karyn Schwartz, and Tricia Neuman. 2021. "Medicare-Covered Older Adults Are Satisfied with Their Coverage, Have Similar Access to Care as Privately-Insured Adults Ages 50 to 64, and Fewer Report Cost-Related Problems." Henry J. Kaiser Family Foundation. May 17. https://www.kff.org/medicare/issue-brief/medicare-covered-older-adults-are-satisfied-with-their-coverage-have-similar-access-to-care-as-privately-insured-adults-ages-50-to-64-and-fewer-report-cost-related-problems/.
3. Gallup. 2013. "Americans Sour on IRS, Rate CDC and FBI Most Positively." Gallup.com. May 23. https://news.gallup.com/poll/162764/americans-views-irs-sharply-negative-2009.aspx.
4. BBC News. 2015. "Why Do Many Americans Mistrust the Federal Reserve?" December 15. https://www.bbc.com/news/business-35079495.
5. Reiss, Dorit. 2020. "Opinion: Free the FDA and the CDC from Political Pressure." CNN. September 4. https://www.cnn.com/2020/09/04/opinions/free-the-fda-and-the-cdc-from-political-pressure-reiss/index.html.
6. Funk, Cary, Meg Hefferon, Brian Kennedy, and Courtney Johnson. 2019. "Trust and Mistrust in Americans' Views of Scientific Experts." August 2. Washington, DC: Pew Research Center. https://www.pewresearch.org/science/2019/08/02/trust-and-mistrust-in-americans-views-of-scientific-experts/.
7. Kiley, Jocelyn. 2018. "Most Continue to Say Ensuring Health Care Coverage is Government's Responsibility." October 3. Washington, DC: Pew Research Center. https://www.pewresearch.org/fact-tank/2018/10/03/most-continue-to-say-ensuring-health-care-coverage-is-governments-responsibility/.
8. AHIP. 2021. "New Research Shows Seniors Are Satisfied with Medigap Coverage." ahip.org. February 25. https://www.ahip.org/new-research-shows-seniors-are-satisfied-with-medigap-coverage/.
9. Kendall, David, Gabriel Horwitz, and Jim Kessler. 2019. "Cost Caps and Coverage for All: How to Make Health Care Universally Affordable." *SSRN*. February 19. https://doi.org/10.2139/ssrn.3356722.
10. Chen, Lanhee J. 2018. "Getting Ready for Health Reform 2020: Republicans' Options for Improving Upon the State Innovation Approach." *Health Affairs* 37 (12): 2076–83. https://doi.org/10.1377/hlthaff.2018.05119.

11. Expanded & Improved Medicare for All Act of 2018, H.R. 676, 115th Congress (2017–2018). https://www.congress.gov/bill/115th-congress/house-bill/676/cosponsors?q=.

12. Berwick, Donald M, Thomas W Nolan, and John Whittington. 2008. "The Triple Aim: Care, Health, and Cost." *Health Affairs (Project Hope)* 27 (3): 759–69. https://doi.org/10.1377/hlthaff.27.3.759.

13. KFF. 2021. "2021 Employer Health Benefits Survey." Henry J. Kaiser Family Foundation. November 10. https://www.kff.org/health-costs/report/2021-employer-health-benefits-survey/.

Chapter 12 Questions Answered

1. Expanded & Improved Medicare for All Act of 2018, H.R. 676, 115th Congress (2017–2018). https://www.congress.gov/bill/115th-congress/house-bill/676/cosponsors?q=.

2. Spatz, Ian. 2018. "IPAB RIP." Health Affairs. February 22. https://www.healthaffairs.org/do/10.1377/hblog20180221.484846/full/.

3. Aaron, Henry J. 2011. "The Independent Payment Advisory Board: Congress's 'Good Deed.'" *New England Journal of Medicine* 364 (25): 2377–79. https://doi.org/10.1056/nejmp1105144.

4. Elmendorf, Douglas. 2010. Letter to Speaker Pelosi, from Congressional Budget Office. March 20. https://www.cbo.gov/sites/default/files/111th-congress-2009-2010/costestimate/amendreconprop.pdf.

5. Oberlander, Jonathan, and Steven B. Spivack. 2018. "Technocratic Dreams, Political Realities: The Rise and Demise of Medicare's Independent Payment Advisory Board." *Journal of Health Politics, Policy and Law* 43 (3): 483–510. https://doi.org/10.1215/03616878-4366196.

6. Brenan, Megan. 2018. "Nurses Again Outpace Other Professions for Honesty, Ethics." Gallup.com. December 20. https://news.gallup.com/poll/245597/nurses-again-outpace-professions-honesty-ethics.aspx.

7. Public Agenda. 2020. "America's Hidden Common Ground on Improving Health Care." February 5. https://www.publicagenda.org/reports/taking-the-pulse-where-americans-agree-on-improving-health-care.

8. KFF. 2019. "Public Opinion on Single-Payer, National Health Plans, and Expanding Access to Medicare Coverage." The Henry J. Kaiser Family Foundation. October 15. https://www.kff.org/slideshow/public-opinion-on-single-payer-national-health-plans-and-expanding-access-to-medicare-coverage/.

63–64, 122, 148; minimal involvement in health care system, 31

federal health care agencies: institutional independence, 148; oversight, 62–63, 156, 157; public opinion of, 147–48. *See also* US Department of Health and Human Services

Federal Insurance Contributions Act (FICA), 126, 131

Federal Open Market Committee (FOMC), 90

Federal Reserve Act, 87, 91, 142, 167

Federal Reserve Bank, 135

Federal Reserve System, as NMB model, 2–3, 45, 60, 61–65, 70, 76–77, 84–93, 110, 133–34, 135, 142, 147–48, 156, 158, 159–60, 163, 164, 167

fee-for-services charges, 50

Flor, Michael, 35

Food and Drug Administration (FDA), 7, 8–9, 19, 20, 24, 53, 62, 76–77, 98, 122, 127, 137, 148, 157

for-profit health care, 11–12, 14, 52, 120, 156. *See also* commercial (private) health insurance; profit motive

government employees, insurance coverage, 111, 125, 143, 152

governments: benefits of EMBRACE for, 110–13, 127. *See also* federal government; state governments

health care administration/administrators, 14–15, 16, 36, 48, 110, 142, 150–51, 152

health care delivery, 24, 40; complexity, 10–15, 27; economic constraints, 84; under NMB, 96; science-based guidelines, 40, 41–42; under single-payer system (HR 676), 156

health care exchange programs, 7–8, 74

health care expenditures, 47–48, 112; for commercial (private) health insurance, 69; under EMBRACE, 125–31, 143; for non-public health care, 128–29; for public health care, 126–28, 130

health care industry, 47–48

Healthcare Information Platform (HIP), 70, 74–76, 96, 119, 129, 130, 136–37, 138; interoperability, 75–76, 104, 119–20, 129;

NMB oversight, 76–77, 79, 90, 93, 97–98, 120, 136, 142; precedents, 81–82, 159–60; Universal Billing Form, 75, 97, 104–5, 117, 120–21, 128–29, 130, 137–38

health care innovations, 31, 40–43; under EMBRACE/NMB, 68, 118–24, 161, 164–65; physician training in, 50, 51; profit motive, 17, 43, 118–19, 122–24. *See also* health care research

health care management agencies, 52–53

health care professionals/providers, 10–12, 50, 165–66; as EMBRACE leadership, 67–68, 141, 142, 148–49, 150, 156, 165–66; impact of EMBRACE on, 99, 104–6; medical-industrial complex and, 49–51, 52; NMB representation, 77, 78, 92, 135–36

health care reform, 2–3, 31, 169; complexity, 1–2, 27–30, 151. *See also* EMBRACE; unified health care system

health care research, 17–23, 27; basic, bench, or clinical, 19–20, 40, 41, 98, 121, 124, 127, 135; EMBRACE and, 119, 122–25; funding, 7, 18, 20, 78; haphazard priorities, 18–20; Healthcare Information Platform and, 76, 121; ineffectual implementation, 20–23; misaligned incentives, 17–18; needs-based, 41–42; NMB oversight, 76–77, 78, 79, 84–85, 90, 127, 135, 136, 137, 157, 162; prioritization, 17, 18–20, 96, 123; translational, 40–41

health care services: basic and supplemental, universal coverage, 32–33, 35, 40; duplication of, 12, 14, 40, 41–42, 63, 112–13, 114, 126–27, 129, 143; prioritization and, 17, 18–24, 80, 84, 86, 120, 162; rationing of, 84

health care system: autonomous profit-making, 7–8; bipartite, 69, 106; complexity of, 27–29, 61, 121–22; evolution of, 6, 24; goals, 17; ineffectiveness and inefficiency of, 1–2, 6; replacement versus reform of, 29–30. *See also* EMBRACE; unified health care system

health care system infrastructure, 67; lack of unified oversight, 1, 6, 8, 16–17, 18–19. *See also* EMBRACE

Health Information Technology for Economic and Clinical Health (HITECH), 138

HEALTH CARE BOOKS FROM HOPKINS PRESS

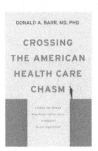 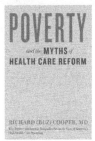 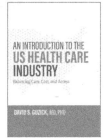 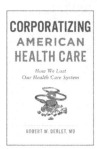 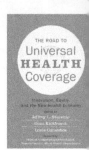

Crossing the American Health Care Chasm

Finding the Path to Bipartisan Collaboration in National Health Care Policy

Donald A. Barr, MD, PhD

"The story of efforts to provide health insurance to the American public from the Truman administration to the present."—Georges C. Benjamin, MD, American Public Health Association

Poverty and the Myths of Health Care Reform

Richard (Buz) Cooper, MD

"A highly sophisticated and powerful analysis of the relationship that exists between poverty and the aggregate cost of health care in this country." —Michael Whitcomb, MD, former Senior Vice President, Association of American Medical Colleges (AAMC)

An Introduction to the US Health Care Industry

Balancing Care, Cost, and Access

David S. Guzick, MD, PhD

"Combining the expert perspective of an economist with that of a hands-on caregiver and senior leader of top health care institutio this unique book should be read by any stude of health care policy."—Eli Y. Adashi, MD, The Warren Alpert Medical School, Brown Univers

Corporatizing American Health Care

How We Lost Our Health Care System

Robert W. Derlet, MD

"This unique book pulls together an excellent review of the crisis in health care and merges it with the author's clinical experience, as we as the lessons he learned as a congressional candidate."—Robert M. Kaplan, Stanford University School of Medicine

The Road to Universal Health Coverage

Innovation, Equity, and the New Health Economy

edited by Jeffrey L. Sturchio, Ilona Kickbusch, and Louis Galambos
foreword by Tedros Adhanom Ghebreyesus, Director-General, World Health Organization

"A refreshingly lucid presentation of the barriers to achieving universal health coverage."—Sir George Alleyne, Director Emeritus, Pan American Health Organization

 @JohnsHopkinsUniversityPress

 @HopkinsPress

 @JHUPress

press.jhu.edu

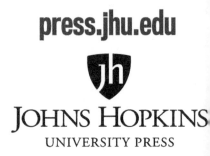